BLADDER CANCER - MANAGEMENT OF NMI AND MUSCLE-INVASIVE CANCER

Edited by **M. Hammad Ather**

Bladder Cancer - Management of NMI and Muscle-Invasive Cancer
http://dx.doi.org/10.5772/63252
Edited by M. Hammad Ather

Contributors

Alejandro Sousa-Escandón, Bulent Erol, Turgay Turan, Asif Yildirim, Turhan Caskurlu, Mustafa Ozan Horsanali, Kutan Ozer, Elena Kiseleva, Natalia Gladkova, Olga Streltzova, Varvara Dudenkova, Anna Maslennikova, Katerina Yunusova, Mikhail Kirillin, Ekaterina Sergeeva, Hosni Khairy Salem, Mariapia Viola-Magni, Samuela Cataldi, Daniela Marocco

Published by InTech

Janeza Trdine 9, 51000 Rijeka, Croatia

Publishing Process Manager Iva Lipovic
Technical Editor SPi Global
Cover InTech Design team

First published April, 2017
Printed in Croatia
Legal deposit, Croatia: National and University Library in Zagreb

Additional hard copies can be obtained from orders@intechopen.com

Bladder Cancer - Management of NMI and Muscle-Invasive Cancer, Edited by M. Hammad Ather
p. cm.
Print ISBN 978-953-51-3077-2
Online ISBN 978-953-51-3078-9

For EU product safety concerns:
IN TECH d.o.o., Prolaz Marije Krucifikse Kozulić 3, 51000 Rijeka, Croatia, info@intechopen.com or visit our website at intechopen.com.

Meet the editor

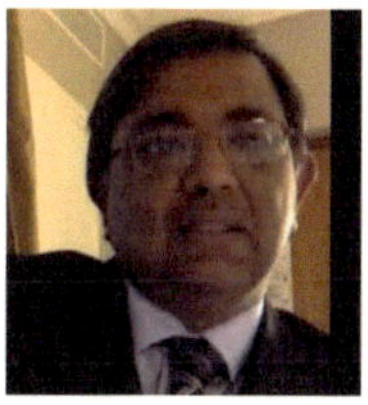

Prof. Hammad Ather is a consultant urological surgeon and head of Urology at the Aga Khan University, Karachi. He is an editorial board member of many international urological journals and author of over 100 articles in international peer-reviewed journals and 10 book chapters. He is also an adviser and reviewer for over two dozen international urological journals. He is also a reviewer for dissertations for various international universities and granting agencies. He has served as the general secretary of Pakistan Association of Urological surgeons (PAUS). He is an international advisory board member of the EULIS (EAU) and national representative of Asia-Pacific Society of Uro-oncology (UAA). His major research and clinical interest is bladder and advanced prostate cancer.

Contents

Preface

The first question that comes to mind when holding this book is why there is a need for another book on bladder cancer (urothelial cancer (UC)). Indeed, it is an extremely widely covered topic in contemporary uro-oncological literature. However, bladder cancer is a major issue both from the standpoint of patients and clinicians. It is considered as one of the most expensive cancers to manage due to frequent and long-term follow-ups needed for non-muscle-invasive (NMI) UC. Cystoscopy is currently the standard of care for the diagnosis and surveillance for NMI UC. Newer diagnostic tools such as urinary markers may assist in a more cost-effective manner in detecting early recurrence of UC of urinary bladder; however, they are not currently validated to replace cystoscopy. The use of photodynamic diagnosis enhances tumor visibility and improves transurethral resection of bladder (TURB) cancer results, potentially reducing recurrence rates and lowering treatment costs. The first section of the book deals with these questions. Authors have tried to assess the contemporary status of these markers.

What makes UC of the bladder a particularly interesting condition is that it exists in two unique forms, i.e., NMI and muscle-invasive (MI) states. They have varied course with low-grade Ta and T1 cancers behaving as a local disease (more like a benign tumor), and, not surprisingly, it is locally treated, whereas MI UC is a potentially lethal disease with very high risk of metastases. The watershed between the two entities is CIS and high-grade NMI.

One of the major concerns in NMI UC of the bladder is recurrence and progression to a higher stage and grade. Up to 30% of NMIBC patients suffer progression to MIBC. In the MI UC of the bladder, the contemporary question of interest is how to reduce mortality in over 50% of appropriately treated patients at 5 years. Two potential strategies to improve outcome are to offer early cystectomy in high-risk NMI UC and offer neoadjuvant and adjuvant chemotherapy in MI UCB. There are limited data on the utility of various clinicopathological markers in the identification of patients who would benefit most from these interventions without risking over treatment. Outcome prediction has improved through the development of nomograms and predictive models; however, there is a dire need of validated molecular markers in identifying patients who would benefit from further interventional treatment. Authors in the first section of the book on NMI UC have focused on the utility of various existing and potential markers for prognosis.

Although some of the non-muscle cancers can progress to muscle-invasive stage, generally these two are considered as separate entities. Most at risk for progression are so-called high-risk cancers according to EORTC risk stratification. However, ~50% of patients diagnosed as high risk in fact do not progress within 3 years. Several markers have been studied to predict the potential of NMI to progress, including microRNAs. Rosenberg and colleagues[1] have studied the role of microRNAs and noted their utility for prognosis in patients with urothelial carcinoma. They noted that the expression levels of several microRNAs, including miR-29c*, identified high- and low-risk groups.

M. Hammad Ather
Aga Khan University
Pakistan

[1]Rosenberg E, Baniel J, Spector Y, Faerman A, Meiri E, Aharonov R, Margel D, Goren Y, Nativ O. Predicting progression of bladder urothelial carcinoma using microRNA expression. BJU Int. 2013 Nov;112(7):1027-34.

Section 1

Non-Muscle-Invasive Urothelial Cancer

Intravesical Treatment Modalities in Bladder Cancer: Current and Future Perspectives

Turgay Turan, Bulent Erol, Asıf Yıldırım and
Turhan Çaşkurlu

Additional information is available at the end of the chapter

http://dx.doi.org/10.5772/66305

Abstract

Non-muscle-invasive bladder cancers encompass the pathological stages of Ta, T1, and carcinoma in situ. To prevent recurrence, intravesical therapy, which is performed after complete transurethral resection, is the current standard therapy for non-muscle-invasive bladder cancers. In patients with low-risk non–muscle-invasive bladder cancer, post-transurethral resection (TUR) management is a single immediate intravesical instillation of chemotherapy alone. For an intermediate-risk patient, a 6-week course of induction intravesical chemotherapy or immunotherapy can be adapted. Bacillus Calmette-Guerin vaccine is still the gold standard of immunomodulating intravesical treatment used to reduce recurrence and progression. Nanotechnology is being developed for the diagnosis and treatment of non-muscle-invasive bladder cancer. The newly developed technology will be able to change intravesical therapy success in non-muscle-invasive bladder cancer.

Keywords: Bacillus Calmette-Guerin, bladder cancer, intravesical chemotherapy, intravesical immunotherapy, nanoparticle

1. Introduction

Bladder cancer (BC) is prevalent in the United States. It was estimated that the number of new bladder cancer cases would reach 76,960 in 2016 [1]. Non-muscle-invasive bladder cancers (NMIBCs) are among the most (75%) newly diagnosed cases [2]. NMIBC encompasses the pathological stages of Ta, T1, and carcinoma in situ (CIS). Patients with low-grade Ta disease have a very low risk of progression. Patients with T1 disease with concurrent CIS have a higher risk of progression and recurrence, approaching 50% [3]. To prevent recurrence, intravesical therapy, which is performed after complete transurethral resection, is the current standard therapy for NMIBC. The risk categorization of the recurrence and progression of NMIBC is based on the European Organization for Research and Treatment of Cancer (EORTC) risk table developed from the data of 2596 patients from seven studies [3]. The scoring system is based on the six most essential clinical and pathologic factors, that is, the number of tumors, tumor size, prior recurrence rate, T category, presence of concurrent CIS, and tumor grade (WHO 1973). Another NMIBC scoring model is the Club Urológico Español de Tratamiento Oncológico (CUETO) model derived from 1062 patients from four trials [4]. As these two

	EAU [7]	**AUA [11]**
Low risk	Primary, solitary Ta, LG/G1, <3 cm, no CIS	Low-grade, solitary Ta _ 3 cm Papillary urothelial neoplasm of low malignant potential
Intermediate risk	All tumors not defined in the 2 adjacent categories (between the categories of low risk and high risk)	Recurrence within 1 year, low-grade Ta Solitary, low-grade Ta >3 cm Low-grade Ta, multifocal High-grade Ta, ≤3 cm Low-grade T1
High risk	Any of the following: T1 tumor HG/G3 tumor CIS Multiple, recurrent, and large (>3 cm) Ta G1G2 tumors (all conditions must be present at this point)	High-grade T1 Any recurrent, high-grade Ta High-grade Ta, >3 cm (or multifocal) Any CIS Any BCG failure in high-grade case Any variant histology Any LVI Any high-grade prostatic urethral involvement

Table 1. The risk stratifications of NMIBC.

	EAU (Update 2016)
Low risk	One immediate instillation of intravesical chemotherapy after TURB.
Intermediate risk	In patients with previous low recurrence rate (less than or equal to 1 recurrence per year) and expected EORTC recurrence score <5, 1 immediate instillation of intravesical chemotherapy after TURB. In all patients, either 1-year full-dose BCG treatment (induction plus weekly instillations for 3 weeks at 3, 6, and 12 months) or instillations of chemotherapy (the optimal schedule is not known) for a maximum of 1 year.
High risk Subgroup of highest-risk tumors • T1G3/HG associated with concurrent bladder CIS, multiple and/or large T1G3/HG and/or recurrent T1G3/HG, T1G3/HG with CIS in the prostatic urethra, unusual histology of urothelial carcinoma, LVI • BCG failures	Intravesical full-dose BCG instillations for 1–3 years or cystectomy. • RC should be considered. In those who refuse RC, intravesical full-dose BCG instillations for 1–3 years. • RC is recommended.

Table 2. Treatment recommendations of EAU guidelines for NMIBC.

models were compared in an independent group of 4689 patients, an overestimated risk of disease progression and recurrence, especially in high-risk patients, was assessed [5]. A new EORTC nomogram, which was based on 1812 patients who underwent 1–3-year Bacillus Calmette-Guerin (BCG) vaccine maintenance, was recently published [6]. The European Association of Urology (EAU) and the American Urological Association (AUA) defined risk groups (**Table 1**). According to the individual risk classification of a patient, intravesical chemotherapy or immunotherapy is recommended according to EAU guidelines (**Table 2**) [7].

In this chapter, we describe the current state and future perspectives of intravesical therapy for NMIBC.

2. Intravesical therapy

2.1. Intravesical chemotherapy

Intravesical treatment is still accepted as the main treatment modality for NMIBC. Though the transurethral resection of bladder tumor (TURB) by itself can absolutely treat a TaT1 tumor, the recurrence of these tumors commonly occurs, and their progression to muscle-invasive BC (MIBC) can be observed. In patients with low-risk NMIBC, therapy is a single intravesical instillation of chemotherapy alone. Immediately, single instillation eradicates circulating tumor cells after TURB and residual tumor cells at the resection site. After TURB, tumor cell implantation should be started within the first few hours. Thus, tumor cells are implanted in the extracellular matrix [8]. To increase the efficacy of single instillation, chemotherapy should be given as soon as possible after TURB, preferably within the first 2 h. All patients in the low- and intermediate-risk groups should have immediate single intravesical chemotherapy if there is no suspicion of bladder perforation or significant bleeding, which requires bladder irrigation. Odden et al. noted that it can cause complications stemming from drug extravasation [9]. Moreover, in the meta-analysis of Sylvester et al., single instillation decreased the 5-year recurrence rate from 59 to 45%. The risk of recurrence was reduced by a single immediate instillation, but there appeared to be no cure in patients with prior recurrence rates of more than one recurrence per year or European Organization for Research and Treatment of Cancer recurrence scores ≥5. The use of mitomycin C (MMC), epirubicin and pirarubicin, for treatment was beneficial [10].

Although a single instillation of intravesical chemotherapy is used for low-risk BC patients, this treatment is inadequate for intermediate-risk disease, and an induction course 3–4 weeks following TURB is recommended according to the guidelines. For an intermediate-risk patient, a 6-week course of induction intravesical chemotherapy or immunotherapy can be adapted [11]. As a result of a meta-analysis of 3703 patients from 11 randomized trials, a highly significant 44% reduction in the odds of recurrence at 1 year in favor of chemotherapy over TURB alone was reported, but the effects on tumor progression have not been determined [12]. The length and frequency of chemotherapy instillations are still being argued. The guidelines do not support treatment >1 year [13]. Controlled urinary pH, reduced urinary excretion, and the balanced intravesical solution of MMC lowered the recurrence rate [12]. A 1-h instillation of MMC was more beneficial than a 30-min instillation, but no efficient comparisons are attainable for 1- and 2-h instillations [14]. With patients from the high-risk group, using microwave-induced hyperthermia or electromotive drug administration (EMDA) can be efficient. Yet, the current evidence is restricted, and both treatment approaches are thought to be experimental [15, 16]. The study of Friedrich et al. included 495 patients with intermediate- and high-risk disease randomized to 6 weeks of MMC alone, 6 weeks of BCG, or 6 weeks of MMC with a 36-month maintenance regime. They reported that maintenance MMC was prevalent at reducing the risk of recurrence when compared to 6 weeks MMC and 6 weeks BCG ($p = 0.001$). They also showed that maintenance MMC was superior to induction BCG in reducing recurrence [17]. However, Hendricksen et al. suggested an immediate instillation with an intensive regime without a maintenance regime [18]. A randomized trial was conducted that compared radio frequency-induced hyperthermic MMC to BCG in 190 intermediate- to high-risk patients treated with 1 year of maintenance treatment. This study showed that 24-month recurrence-free survival (RFS) in patients was definitely better in the hyperthermic MMC arm in per-protocol analysis ($p = 0.008$) [19]. Still, a similarity was found in the complete response rates for CIS between the two groups. The results of this study were hopeful, and hyperthermic MMC can play a major role in the management of high-risk NMIBC in the future. However, no guidelines have advised that the use of device-assisted chemotherapy is not recommended until now. No changes have been made in treatment modalities for intravesical therapy for NMIBC over the past three decades. Gemcitabine and chemohyperthermia (CHT) are options for BCG therapy as adjuvant treatments for intermediate- and high-risk papillary NMIBC, but they are not yet considered standard.

2.2. Intravesical immunotherapy

Intravesical immunotherapy is well known, and its beneficial results for patients suffering from NMIBC are clear. BCG is still the gold standard of immunomodulating intravesical treatment used to reduce recurrence and progression, and its effect on the improvement of tumor-specific survival has been great. A meta-analysis has proved that BCG after TURB is superior to TURB alone or to TURB plus chemotherapy for negating the recurrence of NMIBC [20]. Morales et al. were the first to describe the BCG induction regime of once a week for 6 weeks in 1976. This is still supported today [21]. Many diverse maintenance schedules have been used. However, it is not possible to determine the most effective BCG maintenance schedule [22, 23]. To prevent recurrence or progression, a minimum of 1 year of maintenance BCG is needed to experience the superiority of BCG over MMC [24]. It is not possible to know the optimal number of induction instillations and the optimal frequency and duration of maintenance instillations. EORTC carried out a randomized controlled trial (RCT) of 1355 patients, which indicated that after BCG is given at full dose, 3 years of maintenance decreases the recurrence rate compared with 1 year in high-risk patients, but this is not seen in intermediate-risk patients [25]. In an RCT of 397 patients, CUETO recommended that in high-risk tumors, maintenance with only one instillation every 3 months for 3 years might not be sufficient [26]. In an RCT of 229 patients, a Finnbladder-6 study showed the efficiency of a monthly maintenance-BCG regimen and suggested that it was more beneficial for preventing recurrence than a similar regimen of epirubicin and interferon-α2a [27]. To achieve a reduction in BCG toxicity, the instillation of a reduced dose was to be proposed. The EORTC found no difference in toxicity between one-third and full-dose BCG [28].

BCG instillations can be more beneficial for patients with NMIBC recurrence after a chemotherapy regimen. The continuity of BCG is not appropriate for patients with BCG failure because of a lack of response to therapy; in this case, radical cystectomy is more preferable. Several bladder preservation strategies may be classified as immunotherapy [29], chemotherapy, device-assisted therapy, and combination therapy [30, 31]. In one RCT, unified MMC and BCG reduced recurrences, yet the result of this combination was more toxic compared with that of BCG monotherapy [32]. In another RCT, for frequently recurrent cases of NMIBC, the use of weekly MMC followed by monthly BCG showed a significantly higher rate of efficacy in the reduction of the recurrence rate instead of BCG and interferon [33]. The incomplete BCG instillations due to intolerance prevent the appearance of the best treatment options for patients with high-risk tumors. Non-high-grade recurrence after BCG is not accepted as BCG failure. Treatment techniques should be decided according to tumor characteristics. For EAU, BCG failure is assessed as the development of MIBC, the recurrence of high-grade NMIBC, or pCIS during or after BCG treatment, and cystectomy is advised in these cases [7]. BCG is still considered a cornerstone treatment for high-grade NMIBC; however, the toxicity, limited efficacy in a subset of patients, and recurrence rates show the need for more effective treatment options. Recombinant BCG, monoclonal antibodies, vaccines, and adoptive immunotherapy are alternatives aimed at directing these deficiencies.

2.3. The future of intravesical therapy

To increase the dwell time of intravesical drugs, intravesical drug delivery devices implanted in the bladder are developed and abandoned in place for a length of time. This provides an increase in the drug's exposition period of time in the bladder mucosa.

The lidocaine-releasing intravesical system (LiRIS®) device was advanced as a result of experiments on rabbits. LiRIS has a double-lumen tube. While one of the lumens contains drug tablets, the other consists of lumen superelastic wire. This new technology includes a small flexible osmotic drug pump that provides the release of the drug within 2 weeks. The Massachusetts Institute of Technology by Lee and Cima carried out the research for this device, which demonstrated increased levels of lidocaine in the bladder tissue of rabbits after 3 days of exposure [34, 35]. The current use of this device is for the intravesical delivery of lidocaine in interstitial cystitis patients in phase 2 trials. Its application to bladder cancer treatments will be decided based on the results of future research studies.

A phase 1 trial is designed to deal with the safety and tolerability of the gemcitabine-releasing intravesical system (GemRIS). This system is based on the controlled release of gemcitabine during the 7-day indwelling time. As a consequence of intravesical drug delivery devices, the intravitreal delivery of drugs to the eye is seen as an achievement in the field of ophthalmology [36, 37]. Using similar concepts may bring about success in the development of intravesical drug delivery devices.

2.3.1 Nanotechnology

The treatment of NMIBC nanotechnology is a newly developed technology. Biological and cytotoxic agents for intravesical instillation are some of the therapeutic applications of nanotechnology in NMIBC. The intravesical instillation of live BCG bacteria requires standard care for high-grade NMIBC; however, this treatment has significant side effects, including BCG infections, sepsis, and even death. The harmful components of BCG bacteria have been explored to eradicate live bacteria without any risks. Nakamura et al. enclosed BCG-CWS within 166-nm liposomes, and this formulation showed efficacy in rat models against the development of bladder cancer [38]. The combination of chitosan and polysaccharide-based nanoparticles, chitosan and polylactic acid or chitosan and poly (ε-caprolactone) may be given with mitomycin C, and these nanoparticle drug delivery systems have demonstrated a similar efficacy to that of the release of the pure drugs. This delivery system indicated that the drug was slowly percolated out of the particles. As the polysaccharide structure might play the role of a bioadhesive, a rise in the exposure of the drug to the bladder surface may be observed, even after voiding [39].

The solubility of a drug is increased by nanoparticle albumin bound (NAB) particles to provide conveyance across tumor epithelial cells by interacting with albumin receptors. McKiernan et al. had phase I and II studies with NAB paclitaxel in patients with recurrent NMIBC who especially had failure with one prior BCG regimen. They observed great efficacy and response to this treatment technique in 10 out of 28 (36%) patients [40].

Paclitaxel has also been investigated with gelatin polymer nanoparticles. Lu et al. furthermore demonstrated drug retention in bladder tissue up to 1 week, which means a 360 times higher drug effect on tumor tissue than on normal bladder tissue [41]. The influence of reverse thermosensitive hydrogels has been explored to learn whether they increase the dwell time of intravesical drugs. These polymer hydrogels maintain their liquid character at cold temperatures and turn into gels at body temperature. To serve plenty of urologic uses, Urogen Pharma developed a reverse thermosensitive hydrogel. MMC is in VesiGel™ at a high dose, and this gel is released into the bladder with the help of a Foley catheter. Then, the coating of hydrogen comes out and turns into a solidified gel reservoir. The release of the drug from the gel can increase the dwell time to 6–8 h. The gel dissolves completely and is thrown out of the body via voided urine. According to preclinical results, there is an increased level of MMC in bladder tissue at the same dose of MMC alone, and there is a higher concentration of MMC in the bladder for a longer period of time [42]. Clinical trials are still going on. These also include the prospective optimized instillation of mitomycin for bladder cancer (OPTIMA) study, which will compare the standard intravesical instillation of MMC versus instillation with VesiGel™ prior to TURB in NMIBC. Urogen Pharma MitoGel™, which is developed by Urogen Pharma, uses a ureteral catheter to deliver hydrogel with MMC while treating upper-tract urothelial cancer. Safety and feasibility have been established via preclinical trials [43].

Imiquimod is an immunotherapeutic toll-like receptor 7 (TLR7) agonist. TMX-101 is a liquid formulation of imiquimod. A hydrogel with imiquimod and its safety for intravesical use for pTa and pT1 disease has been established via studies on phase I [44, 45]. A study for phase 2 patients with CIS should be completed soon.

A separate group has conducted another investigation on the use of BackStop Gel®. This treatment consists of a reverse thermosensitive hydrogel from Boston Scientific, which is designed to prevent stone fragment retropulsion during ureteroscopy and to ensure the delivery of MMC to the upper tract of pigs [46]. In the study of Wang et al., MMC was given to the ureters via ureteroscopy, and by closing the system with a thermosensitive polymer plug, MMC was able to stay in the ureters at least 1 h. Then, they recorded the intrarenal pressure and histopathologic differences of the kidney. Finally, they published that the polymer plug was safe [47]. In the study of Tyagi et al., using thermosensitive hydrogel misoprostol on rats significantly reduced urinary frequency with the cyclophosphamide-induced cystitis model [48]. OncoGel (PLGA-PEG-PLGA plus Paclitaxel) was studied in the treatment of esophageal cancer, brain cancer, and other solid tumors [49]. Pluronic F127 is being investigated in other oncologic settings with regard to the effect of its use in combination with nanoparticles to deliver hydrophobic chemotherapeutics in depot fashion [50].

2.3.2. *Mucoadhesives*

Mucoadhesive carriers attach to the bladder epithelium to surrender the dwell time in this treatment technique. Mucoadhesive nanogels were recently analyzed in the porcine urinary bladder and can be a candidate for ensuring the intravesical delivery of hydrophobic drugs in BC therapy [51]. Chitosan, whose investigation is currently being completed, is the main agent. Chitosan enhances the permeability of the urinary bladder wall [52]. Zaharoff et al. evaluated the effect of chitosan/interleukin-12 on a mice bladder cancer model. A preclinical study showed that chitosan/IL-12 had high immune response [53]. Through this therapy, it is possible to decrease the number of intravesical treatments required and the costs of frequent treatment and surveillance. This also shows a novel intravesical for the systemic transfer of immunity with the potential to treat locally advanced or metastatic disease [54]. Through this therapy, it is possible to decrease the number of intravesical treatments required and the costs of frequent treatment and surveillance. In the trial of Zhang et al., the effect of a magnetic chitosan thermosensitive hydrogel in the delivery of BCG in rat bladders was investigated. Benefitting from previously described concepts, they developed a chitosan and Beta-glycerophosphate with a base of thermosensitive hydrogel; it comprised Fe_3O_4 magnetic nanoparticles. They indicated the ongoing release of BCG over 48 h in the presence of a magnetic field. They also showed an increase in the antitumor efficacy of BCG [55]. In addition, a study on chitosan with gemcitabine was conducted [56]. A recent study reported the successful formulation of chitosan and thioglycolic acid nanoparticles that were loaded with gemcitabine and then stayed in chitosan gel or polaxmer hydrogel. The results revealed a great number of losses in the bioadhesive gelling ability of polaxmer. This occurs because it is diluted with an artificial urine solution as compared to chitosan gel.

2.3.3. *Chemohyperthermia, electromotive drug administration, and gemcitabine*

The use of chemohyperthermia and electromotive drug administration was explored to improve the distribution of intravesical therapies in research carried out in 2000. CHT established a connection between intravesical chemotherapy and hyperthermia. The most prevalent chemotherapeutic agent used in CHT is MMC. Some studies with promising results reported a relative reduction in recurrence up to 59% when compared to MMC alone. However, a meta-analysis determined that desperate conclusions could not be declared because of the deficiency of randomized trials and heterogeneous data [15]. EMDA uses the concepts of iontophoresis, electro-osmosis, and electroporation to carry the movement of drugs to the urothelium with an electric current [57]. Di Stasi et al. studied EMDA comprehensively. Their first RCT held in 2003 contained significantly higher response rates at 3 and 6 months for the EMDA-MMC group when compared to the passive diffusion group, as well as a significantly higher peak plasma concentration of MMC following EMDA when compared to passive diffusion [58]. More recently, the combination of BCG and EMDA with MMC was taken into account as a study. However, the significant costs associated with EMDA and its tolerability seem problematic. Therefore, the usage of both CHT and EMDA is not common at this time. According to the EAU guideline on NMIBC, both CHT and EMDA are experimental because of a lack of adequate evidence. Furthermore, the AUA guideline on NMIBC does not recommend their use for the same reason, yet it informs that CHT may be effective for further studies [11]. Neither CHT nor EMDA is accepted for use in the United States. There are ongoing trials to evaluate the use of CHT and EMDA.

Gemcitabine is a nonvesicant chemotherapeutic drug. Skinner et al. reported the results of a phase 3 trial in 2013. The study dealt with 47 patients with two previous BCG failures who each received 2 g of intravesical gemcitabine weekly for 6 weeks of induction, which was followed by monthly maintenance for 1 year. The RFS rate was 28% at 1 year and 21% at 2 years [59]. Until now, only a single study has been carried out that has compared the results of intravesical gemcitabine with those of another agent. In one RCT, Di Lorenzo et al. [60] studied a cohort of patients with a single prior BCG failure. The patients were randomized to receive either twice weekly intravesical gemcitabine for 6 weeks or weekly intravesical BCG for 6 weeks, followed by a 3-week mini-cycle maintenance therapy at 3, 6, and 12 months if disease free. A total of 40 high-risk patients were registered in each arm. After 2 years, the RFS rate in the gemcitabine arm was 19%, and in the BCG arm, it was 3%. Its optimistic tolerability, mild efficacy, and low rate of progression ensure that gemcitabine monotherapy be considered for salvage therapy in select patients.

2.3.4. Photodynamic therapy

Photodynamic therapy (PDT) includes a photo-sensitizing drug that is selectively taken up by malignant cells and followed by the irradiation of these cells with light of a specific wavelength. In 2014, Lee et al. [61] announced their results by using Radachlorin-based PDT for the treatment of high-grade NMIBC that had previously undergone BCG and showed intolerance to BCG or with refractory disease. Patients were checked via cystoscopy and cytology with or without bladder biopsies for the first 3 months and then at 3-month intervals thereafter. All patients were free of tumors at 3 months, and 91, 64.4, and 60.1% of them remained disease free at 12, 24, and 30 months, respectively. Recent reports on the efficacy of a Radachlorin-based protocol and mild side effects are really promising, but the need exists for replication and confirmation before further dissemination.

New clinical trials should be carried out on these nanoformulations and others, especially those covered with cancer-targeting ligand on the surface. These studies can possibly increase the response rate, alleviate recurrence, and decrease the need for cystectomy.

3. Conclusion

Intravesical therapy serves to alleviate the risk of bladder cancer recurrence and progression. Gemcitabine and chemohyperthermia are options for BCG therapy as adjuvant treatment for intermediate- and high-risk papillary NMIBC, but they are not yet considered standard. The newly developed technology will be able to change intravesical therapy success in non-muscle-invasive bladder cancer. New clinical trials should be carried out on nanoformulations, especially those covered with cancer-targeting ligand on the surface, and these studies can possibly increase the response rate, alleviate recurrence, and decrease the need for cystectomy.

Author details

Turgay Turan, Bulent Erol*, Asıf Yıldırım and Turhan Çaşkurlu

*Address all correspondence to: erolbulent@yahoo.com

Istanbul Medeniyet University Faculty of Medicine, Department of Urology, Istanbul, Turkey

References

[1] Siegel RL, Miller KD and Jemal A: Cancer statistics, 2016. CA Cancer J Clin. 2016;66:7–30.

[2] Nielsen ME, Smith AB, Meyer AM, Kuo TM, Tyree S, Kim WY, et al. Trends in stage-specific incidence rates for urothelial carcinoma of the bladder in the United States: 1988 to 2006. Cancer 2014;120(1):86–95.

[3] Sylvester RJ, van der Meijden AP, Oosterlinck W, Witjes JA, Bouffioux C, Denis L, et al. Predicting recurrence and progression in individual patients with stage Ta T1 bladder cancer using EORTC risk tables: a combined analysis of 2596 patients from seven EORTC trials. Eur Urol 2006;49:466–77.

[4] Fernandez-Gomez J, Madero R, Solsona E, Unda M, Martinez-Pineiro L, Gonzalez M, et al. Predicting nonmuscle invasive bladder cancer recurrence and progression in patients treated with bacillus Calmette–Guerin: the CUETO scoring model. J Urol 2009;182:2195–203.

[5] Xylinas E, Kent M, Kluth L, Pycha A, Comploj E, Svatek RS, et al. Accuracy of the EORTC risk tables and of the CUETO scoring model to predict outcomes in nonmuscle invasive urothelial carcinoma of the bladder. Br J Cancer 2013;109:1460–6.

[6] Cambier S, Sylvester RJ, Collette L, Gontero P, Brausi MA, van Andel G, et al. EORTC nomograms and risk groups for predicting recurrence, progression, and disease-specific and overall survival in non-muscle-invasive stage Ta–T1 urothelial bladder cancer patients treated with 1–3 years of maintenance Bacillus Calmette–Guérin. Eur Urol 2016;69:60–9.

[7] Babjuk M, Böhle A, Burger M, Capoun O, Cohen D, Compérat EM, et al. EAU guidelines on non-muscle-invasive urothelial carcinoma of the bladder: Update 2016. Eur Urol 2016 Jun 17. pii: S0302-2838(16)30249-4. doi: 10.1016/j.eururo.2016.05.041. [Epub ahead of print]

[8] Bohle A, Jurczok A, Ardelt P, Wulf T, Ulmer AJ, Jocham D, et al. Inhibition of bladder carcinoma cell adhesion by oligopeptide combinations in vitro and in vivo. J Urol 2002;167:357–63.

[9] Oddens JR, van der Meijden AP, Sylvester R. One immediate postoperative instillation of chemotherapy in low risk Ta,T1 bladder cancer patients. Is it always safe? Eur Urol 2004;46:336–8.

[10] Sylvester RJ, Oosterlinck W, Holmang S, Sydes MR, Birtle A, Gudjonsson S, et al. Systematic review and individual patient data meta-analysis of randomized trials comparing a single immediate instillation of chemotherapy after transurethral resection with transurethral resection alone in patients with stage pTa-pT1 urothelial carcinoma of the bladder: which patients benefit from the instillation? Eur Urol 2016;69:231–44.

[11] Chang SS, Boorjian SA, Chou R, Clark PE, Daneshmand S, Konety BR, et al. Diagnosis and treatment of non-muscle invasive bladder cancer: AUA/SUO guideline. J Urol 2016 Jun 16. pii: S0022-5347(16)30629-2. doi: 10.1016/j.juro.2016.06.049. [Epub ahead of print]

[12] Huncharek M, McGarry R, Kupelnick B. Impact of intravesical chemotherapy on recurrence rate of recurrent superficial transitional cell carcinoma of the bladder: results of a meta-analysis. Anticancer Res 2001;21:765–9.

[13] Sylvester RJ, Oosterlinck W, Witjes JA. The schedule and duration of intravesical chemotherapy in patients with non-muscle invasive bladder cancer: a systematic review of the published results of randomized clinical trials. Eur Urol 2008;53:709–19.

[14] Au JL, Badalament RA, Wientjes MG, Young DC, Warner JA, Venema PL, et al. Methods to improve efficacy of intravesical mitomycin C: results of a randomized phase III trial. J Natl Cancer Inst 2001;93:597–604.

[15] Lammers RJ, Witjes JA, Inman BA, et al. The role of a combined regimen with intravesical chemotherapy and hyperthermia in the management of non–muscle invasive bladder cancer: a systematic review. Eur Urol 2011;60:81–93.

[16] Di Stasi SM, Giannantoni A, Giurioli A, Valenti M, Zampa G, Storti L, et al. Sequential BCG and electromotive mitomycin versus BCG alone for high-risk superficial bladder cancer: a randomised controlled trial. Lancet Oncol 2006;7:43–51.

[17] Friedrich MG, Pichlmeier U, Schwaibold H, Conrad S, Huland H. Long-term intravesical adjuvant chemotherapy further reduces recurrence rate compared with short-term intravesical chemotherapy and short-term therapy with bacillus Calmette–Guérin (BCG) in patients with non-muscle-invasive bladder carcinoma. Eur Urol 2007;52:1123–30.

[18] Hendricksen K, Witjes WP, Idema JG, Kums JJ, van Vierssen Trip OB, de Bruin MJ, et al. Comparison of three schedules of intravesical epirubicin in patients with non-muscle-invasive bladder cancer. Eur Urol 2008;53:984–91.

[19] Arends TJ, Nativ O, Maffezzini M, de Cobelli O, Canepa G, Verweij F, et al. Results of a randomised controlled trial comparing intravesical chemohyperthermia with mitomycin C versus Bacillus Calmette–Guerin for adjuvant treatment of patients with intermediate- and high-risk non-muscle invasive bladder cancer. Eur Urol 2016; 69: 1046–52.

[20] Malmstrom PU, Sylvester RJ, Crawford DE, Friedrich M, Krege S, Rintala E, et al. An individual patient data meta-analysis of the long-term outcome of randomised studies comparing intravesical mitomycin C versus bacillus Calmette-Guerin for non-muscle invasive bladder cancer. Eur Urol 2009;56:247–56.

[21] Morales A, Eidinger D, Bruce AW. Intracavitary Bacillus Calmette–Guerin in the treatment of superficial bladder tumors. J Urol 1976;116:180–3.

[22] Sylvester RJ, van der Meijden A, Lamm DL. Intravesical bacillus Calmette-Guerin reduces the risk of progression in patients with superficial bladder cancer: a meta-analysis of the published results of randomized clinical trials. J Urol 2002;168:1964–70.

[23] Lamm DL, Blumenstein BA, Crissman JD, Montie JE, Gottesman JE, Lowe BA, et al. Maintenance bacillus Calmette-Guerin immunotherapy for recurrent TA, T1 and carcinoma in situ transitional cell carcinoma of the bladder: a randomized Southwest Oncology Group Study. J Urol 2000;163:1124–9.

[24] Bohle A, Bock PR. Intravesical bacille Calmette-Guerin versus mitomycin C in superficial bladder cancer: formal meta-analysis of comparative studies on tumor progression. Urology 2004;63:682–6, discussion 686–7.

[25] Oddens J, Brausi M, Sylvester R, Bono A, van de Beek C, van Andel G, et al. Final results of an EORTC-GU cancers group randomized study of maintenance bacillus Calmette-Guerin in intermediate- and high-risk Ta, T1 papillary carci- noma of the urinary bladder: one-third dose versus full dose and 1 year versus 3 years of maintenance. Eur Urol 2013;63:462–72.

[26] Martinez-Pineiro L, Portillo JA, Fernandez JM, Zabala JA, Cadierno I, Moyano JL, et al. Maintenance therapy with 3-monthly bacillus Calmette-Guerin for 3 years is not superior to standard induction therapy in high-risk non-muscle-invasive urothelial bladder carcinoma: final results of randomised CUETO study 98013. Eur Urol 2015;68:256–62.

[27] Marttila T, Järvinen R, Liukkonen T, Rintala E, Boström P, Seppänen M, et al. Intravesical Bacillus Calmette-Guérin versus combination of epirubicin and interferon-α2a in

reducing recurrence of non-muscle-invasive bladder carcinoma: FinnBladder-6 study. Eur Urol 2016 Aug;70(2):341–7. doi: 10.1016/j.eururo.2016.03.034. Epub 2016 Apr 13.

[28] Brausi M, Oddens J, Sylvester R, Bono A, van de Beek C, van Andel G, et al. Side effects of bacillus Calmette-Guerin (BCG) in the treatment of intermediate- and high-risk Ta, T1 papillary carcinoma of the bladder: results of the EORTC Genito-Urinary Cancers Group randomised phase 3 study comparing one-third dose with full dose and 1 year with 3 years of maintenance BCG. Eur Urol 2014;65:69–76.

[29] Wang Y, Yang M, Yu Q, Yu L, Shao S, Wang X. Recombinant Bacillus Calmette-Guerin in urothelial bladder cancer immunotherapy: Current strategies. Expert Rev Anticancer Ther 2015;15:85–93.

[30] Morales A, Herr H, Steinberg G, Given R, Cohen Z, Amrhein J, et al. Efficacy and safety of MCNA in patients with non-muscle invasive bladder cancer at high risk for recurrence and progression after failed treatment with bacillus Calmette-Guerin. J Urol 2015;193:1135–43.

[31] Yates DR, Brausi MA, Catto JW, Dalbagni G, Rouprêt M, Shariat SF, et al. Treatment options available for bacillus Calmette-Guerin failure in non-muscle invasive bladder cancer. Eur Urol 2012;62:1088–96.

[32] Solsona E, Madero R, Chantada V, Fernandez JM, Zabala JA, Portillo JA, et al. Sequential combination of mitomycin C plus bacillus Calmette-Guerin (BCG) is more effective but more toxic than BCG alone in patients with non-muscle-invasive bladder cancer in intermediate- and high-risk patients: final outcome of CUETO 93009, a randomized prospective trial. Eur Urol 2015;67:508–16.

[33] Jarvinen R, Marttila T, Kaasinen E, Rintala E, Aaltomaa S, Kallio J, et al. Long-term outcome of patients with frequently recurrent non-muscle-invasive bladder carcinoma treated with one perioperative plus four weekly instillations of mitomycin c followed by monthly bacillus Calmette-Guerin (BCG) or alternating BCG and interferon-alpha2b instillations: prospective randomised FinnBladder-4 Study. Eur Urol 2015;68:611–7.

[34] Cima MJ, Lee H, Daniel K, Tanenbaum LM, Mantzavinou A, Spencer KC, et al. Single compartment drug delivery. J Control Release 2014;190:150–71.

[35] Lee HH, Cima MJ. An intravesical device for the sustained delivery of lidocaine to the bladder. J Control Release 2011;149(2):133–9.

[36] Sanborn GE, Anana R, Torti RE, Nightingale SD, Cal SX, Yates B, et al. Sustained-release ganciclovir therapy for treatment of cytomegalovirus retinitis. Use of an intravitreal device. Arch Ophthalmol 1992;110(2):188.

[37] Callanan DG, Jaffe GJ, Martin DF, Pearson PA, Comstock TL. Treatment of posterior uveitis with a fluocinolone acetonide implant: three-year clinical trial results. Arch Ophthalmol 2008;126(9):1191.

[38] Nakamura T, Fukiage M, Higuchi M, Nakaya A, Yano I, Miyazaki J, et al. Nanoparticulation of BCG-CWS for application to bladder cancer therapy. J. Control. Release 2013;176c:44–53.

[39] Bilensoy E, Sarisozen C, Esendağli G, Doğan AL, Aktaş Y, Sen M, et al. Intravesical cationic nanoparticles of chitosan and polycaprolactone for the delivery of Mitomycin C to bladder tumors. Int J Pharm 2009; 371(1–2):170–176.

[40] McKiernan JM, Holder DD, Ghandour RA, Barlow LJ, Ahn JJ, Kates M, et al. Phase II trial of intravesical nanoparticle albumin bound paclitaxel for the treatment of nonmuscle invasive urothelial carcinoma of the bladder after bacillus Calmette-Gucrin treatment failure. J Urol 2014;192(6):1633–8.

[41] Lu ZZ, Yeh TK, Wang J, Chen L, Lyness G, Xin Y, et al. Paclitaxel gelatin nanoparticles for intravesical bladder cancer therapy. J Urol 2011;185(4):1478–83.

[42] Sagiv SP. Great inventions that trick nature, new delivery system optimises bladder cancer treatment by increasing dwell time. ON drug Delivery. 2013. http://www.ondrugdelivery.com/publications/44/TheraCoat.pdf

[43] Meiron M, Chamie K, Lerner SP, Jeshurun M, Hakim G, Schoenberg MP, et al. Mitogel: Optimizing drug delivery to the upper urinary tract a preclinical evaluation. J Urol 2014;191(4):e914.

[44] Falke J, Lammers RJ, Arentsen HC, Ravic M, Possi R, Cornel EB, et al. Results of a phase 1 dose escalation study of intravesical TMX- 101 in patients with nonmuscle invasive bladder cancer. J Urol 2013;189(6):2077–82.

[45] Arends TJ, Lammers RJ, Falke J, van der Heijden AG, Rustighini I, Pozzi R, et al. Pharmacokinetic, pharmacodynamic, and activity evaluation of TMX-101 in a multicenter phase 1 study in patients with papillary non-muscle-invasive bladder cancer. Clin Genitourin Cancer 2015;13(3): 204–9.e2.

[46] Rane AA, Bradoo A, Rao P, Shivde S, Elhilali M, Anjdjar M, et al. The use of a novel reverse thermosensitive polymer to prevent ureteral stone retropulsion during intracorporeal lithotripsy: A randomized, controlled trial. J Urol 2010;183(4):1417–23.

[47] Wang AJ, Goldsmith ZG, Neisius A, Astroza GM, Oredein-McCoy O, Iqbal MW, et al. Increasing dwell time of mitomycin C in the upper tract with a reverse thermosensitive polymer. J Endourol 2013;27(3):288–93.

[48] Tyagi PP, Li Z, Chancellor M, De Groat WC, Yoshimura N, Huang L. Sustained intravesical drug delivery using thermosensitive hydrogel. Pharm Res 2004;21(5):832.

[49] Elstad NL, Fowers KD. OncoGel (ReGel/paclitaxel) clinical applications for a novel paclitaxel delivery system. Adv Drug Deliv Rev 2009;61(10):785–94.

[50] Gou MM, Li X, Dai M, Gong C, Wang X, Xie Y, et al. A novel injectable local hydrophobic drug delivery system: Biodegradable nanoparticles in thermo-sensitive hydrogel. Int J Pharm 2008;359(1-2):228–33.

[51] Lu S, Neoh KG, Kang ET, Mahendran R, Chiong E. Mucoadhesive polyacrylamide nanogel as a potential hydrophobic drug carrier for intravesical bladder cancer therapy. Eur J Pharm Sci. 2015;72:57–69.

[52] Kerec MM, Bogataj M, Veranic P, Mrhar A. Permeability of pig urinary bladder wall: The effect of chitosan and the role of calcium. Eur J Pharm Sci 2005;25(1):113–21.

[53] Zaharoff DA, Hoffman BS, Hooper HB, Benjamin CJ, Khurana KK, Hance KW, et al. Intravesical immunotherapy of superficial bladder cancer with chitosan/interleukin-12. Cancer Res 2009;69(15):6192–9.

[54] Smith SG, Koppolu BP, Ravindranathan S, Kurtz SL, Yang L, Katz MD, et al. Intravesical chitosan/interleukin-12 immunotherapy induces tumor-specific systemic immunity against murine bladder cancer. Cancer Immunol Immunother 2015;64(6):689–96.

[55] Zhang DD, Sun P, Li P, Xue A, Zhang X, Zhang H, et al. A magnetic chitosan hydrogel for sustained and prolonged delivery of Bacillus Calmette-Guerin in the treatment of bladder cancer. Biomaterials 2013;34(38):10258–66.

[56] Şenyiğit ZA, Karavana SY, İlem-Özdemir D, Çaliskan Ç, Waldner C, Şen S, et al. Design and evaluation of an intravesical delivery system for superficial bladder cancer: Preparation of gemcitabine HCl-loaded chitosan-thioglycolic acid nanoparticles and comparison of chitosan/poloxamer gels as carriers. Int J Nanomedicine 2015;10:6493.

[57] Di Stasi SS, Ridel C. Updates in intravesical electromotive drug administration of mitomycin-C for non-muscle invasive bladder cancer. World J Urol 2009;27(3):325–30.

[58] Di Stasi SS, Giannantoni A, Stephen RL, Capelli G, Navarra P, Massoud R, et al. Intravesical electromotive mitomycin C versus passive transport mitomycin C for high risk superficial bladder cancer: A prospective randomized study. J Urol 2003;170(3):777–82.

[59] Skinner EC, Goldman B, Sakr WA, Petrylak DP, Lenz HJ, Lee CT, et al. SWOG S0353: phase II trial of intravesical gemcitabine in patients with nonmuscle invasive bladder cancer and recurrence after 2 prior courses of intravesical Bacillus Calmette-Guerin. J Urol 2013;190:1200–4.

[60] Di Lorenzo G, Perdonà S, Damiano R, Faiella A, Cantiello F, Pignata S, et al. Gemcitabine versus Bacille Calmette-Guerin after initial Bacille Calmette-Guerin failure in non-muscle-invasive bladder cancer: a multicenter prospective randomized trial. Cancer 2010;116:1893–900.

[61] Lee JY, Diaz RR, Cho KS, Lim MS, Chung JS, Kim WT, et al. Efficacy and safety of photodynamic therapy for recurrent, high grade non muscle invasive bladder cancer refractory or intolerant to Bacille Calmette-Guerin immunotherapy. J Urol 2013;190:1192–9.

Chapter 2

Intravesical Chemohyperthermia for NMIBC: Rationale and Results of This Developing Treatment

Sousa-Escandón Manuel Alejandro,
Flores Carbajal Javier, Sousa-González Daniel and
Rodriguez Gómez Silvia

Additional information is available at the end of the chapter

http://dx.doi.org/10.5772/67280

Abstract

Bladder cancer is the fourth most common cancer in men, and the lifetime risk of getting bladder cancer is 2.4%. Approximately 75% of newly diagnosed cases of bladder cancer are non-muscle-invasive bladder cancer (NMIBC), and half of them will show recurrence and/or progression after transurethral resection. Therefore, after transurethral resection, in high-risk patients, intravesical therapy is mandatory. However, bacillus Calmette-Guérin (BCG) is associated with important side effects such as systemic tuberculosis and bladder retraction. Chemohyperthermia (CHT) has shown a 60% lower recurrence rate than standard mitomycin C (MMC). However, its effectiveness in high-risk patients, especially CIS and BCG refractory patients, is even more important. CHT will probably be an option for patients unsuitable for radical cystectomy or those on whom BCG can't be used. Two main technologies are currently available for intravesical CHT: microwaves and recirculating heated fluids. Both of them have pros and cons that should be known and evaluated by a urologist. In this chapter, we will speak about rationale, technical options, clinical results, ongoing studies, and future perspective for this interesting treatment option for intermediate and high-risk patients with NMIBC.

Keywords: NMIBC, MMC, BCG, chemohyperthermia, radio frequency, recirculant systems, adjuvant, neoadjuvant

1. Background

In 2002, the world-adjusted incidence rate of bladder cancer was 33 new cases/100,000 inhabitants/year. That makes it the fourth tumor with the highest incidence in men, after lung, prostate, and colorectal cancers [1].

Each body tumor has unique characteristics in terms of its presentation, histological types, surgical approaches, and sensitivity to different types of treatment (surgery, chemotherapy, radiotherapy).

Approximately, 95% of bladder neoplasms are urothelial carcinomas, and 75% of them will be diagnosed as non-muscle-invasive tumors. However, they have a high tendency to recur, and one-third of them will reappear during the first 5 years after transurethral resection. Incidence of recurrence and progression is directly related to the tumoral grade and stage, being higher in carcinoma in situ and T1G3 tumors.

Most recidives have similar grade and stage to the original tumor. However, a significant number of bladder cancers progress to invasive tumors whose prognosis and treatment are completely different. Therefore, intravesical postoperative therapy is mandatory, especially in those with medium and high-risk tumors.

The urethra allows ease of access from the outside, which generally allows a resection of the tumor and the application of chemo- and/or immunotherapy locally with minimal systemic toxicity.

Intravesical chemotherapy, *with single postoperative or with maintenance protocols*, is the usual treatment for patients with low and intermediate risk of non-muscle-invasive bladder cancers (NMIBCs). Their side effects are well tolerated, but there is general consensus that chemotherapy is effective in reducing short-term risk for recurrence, but its efficacy is only marginal in the long term [2].

On the other hand, immunotherapy with bacillus Calmette-Guérin (BCG) is the gold standard treatment for high-risk patients. However, BCG is associated with important side effects such as systemic tuberculosis and bladder retraction [3]. Moreover, in the recent past, there has been a limited availability of BCG, which has made us change our old protocols for new ones using a lower dose or reducing the number of instillations. Clearly, there is a scope to optimize and improve current intravesical chemotherapy.

Many new treatment approaches are being researched to increase the effectiveness of adjuvant intravesical therapy. One of the developing treatments for high-risk NMIBC is the combination of intravesical chemotherapy and hyperthermia, called chemohyperthermia (CHT).

Chemotherapy combined with thermal energy has proven higher anticancer activity than chemotherapeutic instillation alone at diminishing recurrence rates. It also appears to improve the bladder preservation rate. Moreover, in the future, CHT may become a standard therapy for high-risk patients with recurrent tumors, for patients who are unsuitable for radical cystectomy, and in cases for which BCG is contraindicated [4].

In this chapter, we will speak about rationale, technical options, clinical results, ongoing studies, and future perspective for this interesting option of treatment for intermediate and high-risk patients with NMIBC.

2. Intravesical therapies for the treatment of NMIBC

2.1. Historical review

The first intravesical treatments can probably be traced to the eleventh century. In the third book of his treatise *Canon of Medicine*, Avicenna described how to inject a list of drugs into the bladder through a hollow cylindrical instrument [5].

The first description of specific intravesical treatment for bladder cancer was carried out in the 1950s by Walton and Sinclair [6]. In the following years, radioactive solutions of sodium bromide and colloidal gold were used with relative success but also important complications.

Jones and Swinney [7] described in 1961 the use of intravesical thiotepa which was later the first intravesical drug FDA approved for NMIBC; however, its side effect rates were high, so it was not commonly used.

Mitomycin C (MMC) is a cross-linking agent that inhibits DNA synthesis, which was discovered by Wataki et al. [8] in 1962. Seven years later, Ogawa [9] instillated MMC simultaneously with radioactive phosphorus, but its toxicity was high. In the following year, Shida et al. [10] published the first results by using intravesical MMC. Almost a decade went by before Kaufman et al. [11] began using it in the USA who was followed a few years later by German urologists. Due to its high molecular weight (329 kDa), there is reduced risk of transurothelial absorption, and side effects are minimal [2].

In 1976, Morales et al. [12] demonstrated the power of immunotherapy to treat bladder cancer by showing BCG effectiveness in patients with carcinoma in situ. Both treatments, chemotherapy with MMC and immunotherapy with BCG, became the gold standard of intravesical therapy for low-medium and high-risk patients, respectively.

Many other drugs and immunotherapeutic agents have been tried against NMIBC in the last half century, but intravesical chemotherapy with MMC remains the most widely used worldwide. However, the reduction of tumoral recurrences is not very high, and even this small difference is lost after 2 years of follow-up, and tumoral progression is not reduced [2].

2.2. What limits the effectiveness of intravesical chemotherapy?

From the evolutionary point of view, the urinary bladder appeared in amphibians as a reservoir to store urine with intention of using it for osmotic regulation of the body by reabsorbing water and sodium in the case of dehydration. However, mammals have an impermeable bladder used as a simple urine reservoir which allows them to eliminate it only a few times a day. Thus, the animal would seek a convenient time to expel it, rather than eliminate it continuously, thereby avoiding the creation of an odorous trail that could be traced by possible predators [13].

Urine contains urea and other toxic substances which have been removed from the bloodstream by the kidney. If they were newly reabsorbed by the bladder, it would be a serious problem to the body. For this reason, the bladder of higher animals has evolved as an almost completely waterproof bag which is also resistant to toxic chemicals present in it.

This is achieved through four fundamental mechanisms [14, 15]. First, the turnover of the urothelium is the slowest of all epithelia in the body. After the division of basal cells, the urothelial cells need 200 days to progress before flaking into the bladder. Due to this slowness in cell division, urothelial cells rarely enter mitosis, and therefore its DNA is less exposed to intravesical toxins. Second, there are some specialized cells called "umbrella" on the endoluminal surface, which have lateral interdigitations and proteins called "uroplakins." Both structures keep umbrella cells intimately connected to their neighbors in an almost completely waterproof way. Third, urothelial cells possess surface structures called "asymmetric unit membrane" (AUM) in both lumen and intraepithelial cells. AUM works as membrane-binding sites for cytoplasmic microfilaments. Its intraepithelial location and association with microfilaments support the hypothesis that AUM has a mechanical function and modulates the surface area of the cell during the relaxation-contraction cycle of the urinary bladder maintaining tightness even at the time of maximum dilatation [16]. And fourth, to help strengthen the sealing, the endoluminal surface of the bladder is covered by a thick layer of negatively charged glycosaminoglycans. This charge is responsible for the electrical rejection of many compounds present in urine and whose resorption would be toxic to the body.

Low absorption of the MMC is not due solely to the waterproof properties of the bladder wall but also to the characteristics of the drug. The MMC is a high molecular weight molecule (*334* Dalton), with a weak negative charge and a relatively hydrophobic behavior. These features make absorption through the urothelium less than 3% of the amount instilled which severely limits its effectiveness [2].

Pharmacokinetic studies [17–19] have shown that systemic absorption of the MMC does not reach significant plasma levels. Average of MMC plasma concentration on patients treated after urothelium recovery was 5.24 ng/mL. Conversely, absorption of MMC instilled immediately after TUR reaches an average of 50 ng/mL, which varies significantly with the resected surface of the bladder mucosa ($p < 0.026$). However, even given immediately after TUR, the MMC fails to achieve the minimum accepted as myelotoxic dose of around 400 ng/mL.

2.3. Why does NMIBC recur so often?

Urothelial bladder carcinoma appears in the form of two main phenotypic variants. The most frequent (80%) is papillary tumors of medium or low grade. Of these, 33–70% will reappear in the first 5 years and 4–9% progress to invasive disease. By contrast, 20% of urothelial carcinomas are high grade (T1-GIII or carcinoma in situ). Of these, one 68–80% will relapse in the first 3 years and, 13–23% will progress to invasive disease [20].

It is important to know what are the mechanisms of recurrence are to try to reduce them. It is thought that there are a total of four mechanisms potentially involved.

The first and clearest is incomplete tumor resection (*evidence level 1*). Its incidence is clearly related to the quality of TURB performed. According to the guidelines of the European Association of Urology, when performing a re-TUR in patients with T1 tumors, 33–53% have residual tumor, and 10% presented infiltrative tumors (T2) after the second TUR-B [20].

In some publications, the numbers of residual tumor reach a high of 78%, and 25–40% of cases will be restaged to more advanced tumors [21]; the surgical methodology of these centers must be reviewed.

In 2006, Divrik et al. [22] compared the efficacy of TUR-B + 8 weeks of MMC (Group 1:68 pts) vs the second TUR-B + 8 weeks of MMC (Group 2:74 pts) in patients with T1 bladder carcinoma achieving significant differences. Disease-free survival at 1 and 3 years was 47 and 37% for Group 1 vs 86 and 68% for Group 2. Recurrences of GII and GIII were 64 and 90% for Group 1 vs 25 and 60% for Group 2. Finally, they observed progression in 11.7% of Group 1 vs 4% in Group 2.

Based on recurrence-free survival as well as the grade and stage of the tumors relapsed, they concluded that recurrences are due to residual tumor and that intravesical chemotherapy post-TUR-B does not compensate inadequate tumor resection.

The second mechanism is the reimplantation of circulating tumor cells that are released during the TUR-B. This process was demonstrated by Soloway et al. [23] by introducing transplantable tumor cells (1×10^6) in the bladder of 50 mice of which half had part of the urothelium electrocoagulated, while the other half did not. Tumoral implants occurred in 54% of mice with burned bladder mucosa, while it appeared in only 12% of those with an intact bladder ($p < 0.005$). They further showed that immediate intravesical MMC, thiotepa, and cisplatin significantly reduced the occurrence of tumoral implants.

The first clinical use of this principle was made by Solsona et al. [24, 25] who administered a dose of MMC within the first 24 hours post-TUR-B and found a decrease in the number of relapses at 2 years in patients with low-risk tumors.

Numerous studies to date have demonstrated its usefulness in significantly reducing tumor recurrence in the first year, regardless of maintenance treatment during this time whether preformed [26] or not [27] ($p < 0.02$). One-year recurrences with immediate instillation ranged from 3.2 to 11.3%, while in the control group ranged between 18.7 and 29%. Although differences persist within 2–3 years, they are not significant statistically [25–27]. A recent meta-analysis quantified the effect on a 1.35 absolute reduction of relapses and the need to treat 7.2 patients to prevent recurrence [28]. However, the main problem with the immediate postoperative instillation is the severe side effects, which may appear if MMC reaches the bladder fat and surrounding organs, which would have devastating consequences [29].

The third cause of relapse is the possible growth of small preexisting microscopic lesions (*which cannot be considered insufficient resections*) originating around the initial tumor and which share genetic characteristics with the original tumor; this area is called *preneoplastic urothelial plate* (*PUP*). The first recurrence seen on patients treated with immediate MMC post-TUR-B appears at 40 months and does so four times more frequently in the area of the previous tumor, in other words, arising from the same PUP [30].

Finally, recurrences may appear years later, by gradual malignization of other dysplastic areas. In fact, first tumoral recidives are four times more frequent in a neighboring area of the original tumor, while only 13% are multifocal. However, from the sixth recurrence, 100% of tumors are multifocal [30]. Once this point is achieved, there are significant clinical implications, which have to be taken into account when choosing patient treatment [31].

PUP theory is based on studies of different vesical urothelial clones by inactivation of chromosome X. This investigation showed that the bladder is lined with a mosaic made up of numerous clones, which are derived from a single stem cell. Each bladder contains about 200–300 patches of 1–2 cm^2. There are usually preexisting genetic alterations in most urothelial tumors, usually located in chromosome 9. Some toxins act by inducing additional genetic changes in the carcinogenesis step process until you get to a point where abnormal cell proliferation is initiated then a hyperplastic epithelium that can develop into cancer in one or more PUP [32].

MMC instillation with extended maintenance has been shown to reduce the number of tumor recurrence in intermediate-risk patients. However, this treatment has no effect on tumoral progression and global survival [33, 34]. Moreover, comparative studies between MMC and BCG have shown that BCG is clearly superior in intermediate and high-risk tumors [33, 34]. To explain this data, we must understand the pathophysiology and pharmacokinetics of MMC applied within the bladder.

3. What is antineoplastic hyperthermia?

Also called thermotherapy, it is a type of therapy for tumors in which the whole body, or part thereof, is subjected to high temperatures (up to 45°C). Numerous studies have shown that high temperatures damage and kill cancer cells by denaturation of their proteins and by preventing DNA repair. However, hyperthermia causes little damage to normal tissue [35, 36].

The first clinical experiences in the use of hyperthermia as a treatment for cancer were performed by Coley [37] more than a century ago. He injected bacterial toxins of *Streptococcus erysipelas* and *Bacillus prodigiosus* with the intention of producing fever. He supposed that fever would activate the immune system and heal a patient with an inoperable sarcoma.

Hyperthermia is almost always used with other forms of treatment for cancer [35, 38]. Numerous studies have shown that hyperthermia makes cancer cells more sensitive to radiation and chemotherapy. These studies have been conducted on different cancers such as sarcoma, melanoma, and cancers of the bladder, brain, breast, cervix, esophagus, lung, rectum, and peritoneal metastases [35, 38–43].

Hyperthermia may be applied in different ways such as to the entire body (*whole body*), regional, intracavitary, local, and interstitial. Similarly, sources of heat are varied and include microwaves, ultrasound, radio frequency, and recirculating liquid systems.

In the case of bladder tumors, there are two types. The first, used in infiltrating cancers, involves the application of external heat on the entire pelvis associating radio- or chemotherapy [42].

The second, used in NMIBC, consists of the intravesical application of heat through microwaves or recirculation of heated liquids. In this type of treatment, a chemotherapeutic agent is associated to the heat in order to achieve a synergistic effect by using both treatments together, which is known as CHT [40, 42].

3.1. Mechanism of action of antineoplastic hyperthermia

The human body has several independent mechanisms to regulate its temperature within appropriate ranges for an adequate function of all its organs. They include vasodilation plus sweating against heat and by body tremors plus vasoconstriction against cold [44]. The body's metabolic processes serve as the main sources of internal heat generation.

The normal thermoregulatory response begins when sensory receptors on the surface of the skin or organs of the core body are activated depending on their temperature thresholds. The information is integrated along their way to the hypothalamus, the main thermoregulatory center. The efferent thermoregulatory answer of the hypothalamus is sent to effector organs of the body to trigger a response able to recover thermic homeostasis [44, 45]. Clinical effects produced by antitumoral hyperthermia are summarized in **Table 1**.

Temperature range	Direct cytotoxic effects	Immune effects	Vascular effects	Others
39–41°C 41–43°C	Slight growth arrest Reversible growth arrest - Mainly in phases M and S - Brief RNA synthesis impaired - Prolonged DNA synthesis impaired	Initial increase intracellular HSP followed by increase of extracellular HSP - Signals to immune cells - Cross priming of CD8+ T cells - Dendritic cell activation - Natural killer activation - Increase cytocine release (IL-6, IL-10)	Vasodilatation which means: Improved tumor blood flow - Improved tissular O2 - Reduced acidosis - Improved drug absorption	Increased drug delivery Increased drug solubility Increased efficacy of many chemotherapeutic drugs - MMC - Gemcitabine - Cisplatin - Cyclophosphamide - Doxorubicin
43–45°C	Irreversible growth arrest - Permanent protein denaturalization - DNA repair impaired - Activation of both apoptotic routes	Altered cytocine production Inactivation of immune cells Reduced expression of extracellular HSP	Reduced tumor blood flow due to vascular collapse - Microthrombosis - Endothelial cell damage - Vessel permeation - Increased acidosis and reduced tissular O2	

Table 1. Action mechanism of chemohyperthermia in NMIBC.

3.1.1. *Direct cytotoxic effects of hyperthermia*

Hyperthermia has cytotoxic effects on tumor cells by means of several mechanisms, including improved antitumoral immunity by direct cytotoxic effects.

The first phase of direct death is characterized by stopping the linear growth, characterized by decreased synthesis of RNA (*short*) and DNA (*prolonged*) specifically in the S phase but also slowing the M phase of the cellular cycle [36, 45–47]. The G1 and G2 phases are relatively protected due to the temperature-dependent expression of heat shock proteins (HSPs) [48]. Tumoral cells reached a state of rapid division circumventing the apoptotic pathways and avoiding the normal detention mechanisms of the cell cycle. If the cell division speed is turned down, this would allow apoptotic mechanisms to kill tumoral cells. During this phase direct cytotoxicity occurs between 41 and 43°C and is reversible after heat removal.

In addition, heat interferes with the ability of the cell to repair damaged proteins produced as a result of chemotherapy or radiotherapy. It is believed that these proteins play a key role in the activation of apoptotic pathways. Deficiencies in DNA repair mechanisms become evident only at 40°C and continue to worsen when temperatures are higher [49]. Above 43°C, an exponential and irreversible growth arrest occurs, and its intensity is dose and time dependant [50]. This phase is characterized by disruption of the cell membrane and denaturation of cellular and transmembrane proteins, distortion of cellular architecture, and ultimately activation of apoptotic and necrotic pathways.

3.1.2. Antitumoral immune response to hyperthermia

The body's ability to use temperatures within the range of fever (39–41°C) to enhance immune system function against infection is well documented [51]. Activation state of the immune system depends on degree and duration of the applied heat [52]. However, we can only subject the patient to temperatures achievable with fever, those which are achievable in vivo. Dendritic cells, natural killer (NK) cells, and phagocytes that play a key role in antitumoral immune mechanisms are directly activated by hyperthermia. HSPs are chaperone tumor-related antigens that can be released or become apparent on the tumoral surface as a result of chemotherapy, radiation, or heat [53].

These HSPs act as stimulating antigens for dendritic cells [54, 55]. Then, these dendritic cells present tumoral antigens to macrophages and T cytotoxic cells CD8+ leading to the release of pro-inflammatory and proapoptotic cytokines that increase tumoral cell destruction [54–56].

When in the extracellular space, HSPs bind to cancer cells' surface to help identify them for cells of the immune system [52]. Increased expression of intercellular adhesion molecules (ICAM) resulting from hyperthermia also leads to increased lymphocyte trafficking to sites where tumoral antigens are present, helping adaptive response against cancer cells [57]. Furthermore, hyperthermia activates the innate immune system by improving the ability of NK cells to destroy tumoral cells [58].

In vitro temperatures above 43°C may cause paradoxical immune responses to the aforementioned, but these responses are less interesting biologically since such high temperatures are difficult to reach and maintain in vivo [54]. While hyperthermia has been shown to enhance the efficacy of immunotherapy in a murine model of pulmonar metastasis [59], this combination has not yet been studied in bladder cancer.

3.1.3. *Vascular effects of hyperthermia*

These effects are variable depending on the intensity of heat and the characteristics of the supplying vascularization. One of the first demonstrations of hyperthermia is vasodilation, which leads to an increase in blood supply to the tumor [60]. This effect enhances the tumor microenvironment for the action of the immune system by improving oxygenation and reducing acidosis [61]. The vasodilation effect is produced with temperature up until about 43°C, above which perfusion will decrease because of vascular collapse; this affects reoxygenation and drug delivery, complicating the empirical formulation of a thermal dose.

In renal tumors, vasodilation has shown an effect of "washing" of the chemotherapeutic and temperature reduction by increasing blood flow at 37°C. However, at the bladder urothelium, the caliber of the blood vessels is small, and its effects by washing the chemotherapeutic or reducing applied heat are very small.

With sustained high temperatures, the opposite effect occurs due to direct endothelial cell damage to the tumoral supplying vessels [62]. These vessels begin to present microvascular thrombosis with consequent decrease in blood flow that leads to the death of tumor cells by hypoxia.

Animal studies performed by Haas et al. [63] showed that hyperthermia alone reduced growth of implanted tumors. However, when administered simultaneously with chemotherapeutic agents its treatment effect increases in a significant way.

Similarly, Van der Heijden et al. [64] showed that chemotherapy and hyperthermia show a synergistic effect increasing the cytotoxicity of epirubicin, EO9, gemcitabine, and MMC. Also, they showed a significant synergy of heat and MMC against four bladder tumoral cell lines [64, 65].

3.1.4. *Increased absorption of MMC by heat*

Dalton et al. [18] studied that the pharmacokinetics of intravesical MMC observing the absorption thereof is significantly affected by dilution, urinary pH, and exposure time. They observed that, with passive instillations, the absorption of the administered dose is less than 30%.

In 2001, Paroni et al. [66] showed that microwave-induced hyperthermia increased MMC absorption, at 30, 45, and 60 min, significantly ($p < 0.008$). However, even higher plasma concentrations achieved with CHT (67 ng/mL), were six times lower than those needed to be myelosuppressive (approx. 400 ng/mL). Similar results were seen by Milla et al. [67] when causing hyperthermia by using recirculating heat liquids.

It is important to understand that increased MMC absorption is not only due to increased permeability of the bladder urothelium but also due to a significant increase in solubility. At 25°C the maximum concentration that we may get by dissolving 1 gr of MMC is 0.8 mg/mL. However, at 40°C, MMC concentrations up to 1.7 mg/mL can be reached when dissolving the same amount of it. (Data from *Kyowa Hakko Co Ltd.*).

3.2. Adjuvant CHT treatment (after TUR-B)

3.2.1. Clinical outcomes: tumoral recurrences

In 2011, a meta-analysis which was composed of a total of 22 studies showed a 59% reduction in tumor recurrences in the group chemohyperthermia against the MMC [4].

T1G3 and CIS tumors subgroup treated with CHT showed greater differences compared to the MMC at normal temperature were patients with T1G3 and CIS tumors. Witjes et al. [68] observed that 92% of patients treated with CHT showed complete eradication of the tumor and only 50% had recurrence after 30 months of follow-up.

Similar results were seen with conductive heat technology; our group found [69] a recurrence-free disease rate of 87.5% in high-risk patients treated with combat recirculant CHT and followed during 2 years. However, Ekin et al. [70] showed that the recurrence-free rates of high-risk patients treated with BWT recirculant CHT were 82 and 61% at 1 and 2 years of follow-up

The first randomized trial comparing CHT vs BCG was published by Arends et al. [71]. They observed a recurrence-free survival after 2 years of follow-up of 78% in the CHT group vs 64.8% with BCG ($p < 0.0082$). Progression was lower than 2% in both groups (p = ns). On the other hand, Ekin et al. [72] concluded that CHT was not as effective treatment as BCG in high-risk NMIBC patients who are BCG naive. The 2-year recurrence-free interval in CHT and BCG groups was 76.2 and 93.9%, respectively, ($p = 0.02$). However, it was a retrospective propensity score-matched study to compare the efficacy of BCG and chemohyperthermia.

Some studies have shown a long-term effect of treatment with CHT. Colombo et al. [73] published results of 65 NMIBC medium-high risk patients treated with CHT or standard MMC and they found that disease-free survival at 10 years was 53% in the group CHT compared to 15% with standard MMC ($p < 0.001$).

Probably, the most important conclusion of the mentioned meta-analysis [4], *and which seems to be confirmed with all subsequently published studies*, is that in the future, the CHT may become a standard treatment for high-risk patients with recurrent tumors that are unfit for radical cystectomy or when BCG treatment is contraindicated.

3.2.2. Tumoral progression after CHT and bladder preservation rates

Lammers et al. [4] also noted that only 0–8% of patients had tumor progression and although this figure is lower than that observed with standard MMC, follow-up duration was too short and cannot draw definitive conclusions.

The survival of patients who failed intravesical therapy and progress to muscle-invasive disease is worse than that of those with NMIBC from the time of diagnosis. Schrier et al. [74] found a cancer-specific survival at 3 years of 37% for patients who progressed to NMIBC, compared to 67% achieved by patients who originally showed with infiltrative tumors. These results were also confirmed by Guzzo et al. [75].

Several studies have investigated the role of CHT in the rescue NMIBC that has not responded to other intravesical treatments. Ayres et al. [76] prospectively evaluated 38 high-risk patients who had failed after BCG and were treated with CHT and found a 50% survival-free disease at 2 years which is a significant success rate for these kinds of patients.

Some comparative studies between BCG failure patients and non-previously treated patients showed better results in the former group. The interim analysis of the Lombardia project (*unpublished data from R. Colombo, Milan, Italy*) showed that, after two years of follow-up, the recurrence-free rates of patients treated with de novo CHT were significantly better than those who had previously failed intravesical treatment (91 and 62%, respectively, $p < 0.006$). Similarly, Van der Heijden et al. [77] followed 76 patients treated with CHT for 2 years, observing a 42% recurrence in the group with a previous failed BCG treatment compared to a 24% recurrence rate in the de novo treatment group.

However, others like Witjes et al. [78] observed no difference in the response rate among patients who had failed BCG and those without ($p = 0.63$). Similarly, Halachmi et al. [79] did not observe any difference in the rate of recurrence at 4 years among those who had failed BCG and those without (46 vs 44%, respectively, $p = 0.54$).

Overall, although the results of CHT in patients who have failed prior to other intravesical regimens are heterogeneous, the truth is that they managed to rescue a significant number of failures after BCG with CHT which is a major advantage of this treatment regimen.

The overall rate of bladder preservation after CHT was 87.6% compared to 79% for MMC (p = ns). Of the 357 patients in all studies, only 38 patients (10.6%) underwent radical cystectomy. Eleven cases (3.1%) were due to tumor progression, other 25 cases (7.0%) due to a high incidence of recurrences, and other 2 cases ($p < 0.006\%$) because of bladder retraction or miction worsening [4].

Similar data were published by Moskovitz et al. [80], with 72% free of recurrence and only 4.7% progression rate in patients who received adjuvant treatment with CHT.

A sequential treatment study using intravesical BCG and CHT was performed in Leicester, UK, to treat 33 high-risk NMIBC patients (*including 40% with Cis*) who were followed during a median of 16 months [81]. Three of them (9%) did not respond and were proposed for radical cystectomy. Two (6%) showed tumoral progression and were treated with radiotherapy. The other 85% of them were disease-free after follow-up.

3.3. Neoadjuvant CHT treatment (before TUR-B)

The rationale about neoadjuvant CHT is based on three main ideas. First, all published data seems to support the idea that apoptotic tumoral cells destroyed by the neoadjuvant CHT treatment stimulate the immune response against them acting as a vaccine against cancer. Second, in patients with tumors unable to be resected with only one TUR-B, Neoadjuvant CHT could diminish number and/or size of tumoral implants avoiding need of a second surgery, this treatment could offer both a more effective treatment and better value for the health-care provider, as they might not need a second TUR-B. Third, many early recurrences are based on growth of minimal tumoral implants which were not seen during surgery and that neoadjuvant CHT is able to eliminate.

Colombo et al. [82] evaluated for the first time the clinical efficacy of neoadjuvant CHT in bladder cancer in 1998. In that study, a total of 19 patients who had tumors that were unresectable in one surgical time or a radical cystectomy was indicated due to its extension. After 8 weekly doses of CHT, the TUR-B was possible in just one surgical time in 16 patients (84%). The histological examination of the sample showed a 47% complete response (CR) and 37% partial response (PR). A radical cystectomy was performed in the remaining three patients because of the extent of the residual tumor. After an average of 33 months of follow-up, eight superficial recurrences were seen, and TUR-B was easily performed without having to remove the bladder.

In 2012, Moskovitz et al. [80] documented a 79% CR rate in a group of patients undergoing neoadjuvant CHT. But what is even more interesting is that 84% of those patients with complete response remained free of recurrence during the follow-up period and the 24% who recurred had TaG1 tumors.

It is important to mention that we do not know that CHT regime is more effective and less toxic. A phase 2 study of Colombo et al. [83] evaluated two CHT protocols including 27 patients each with 40 mg of MMC. Group A received a single weekly dose of MMC (40 mgrs) × 6 weeks, and Group B received 3 weekly doses of MMC (40 mgrs) × 2 months. A 7.4% of patients from Group B did not complete the treatment because of severe urinary local irritative symptoms; other side effects were similar in both groups. However, success rates of both groups were significantly different; histopathological examination of the TUR-B samples showed that only 44.4% of patients from Group A had CR, while 70.4% of Group B patients were free of tumor ($p = 0.04$)

Another study compared the recurrence rate at 5 years among patients who had received more or less than eight doses of CHT in a neoadjuvant setting. While the group receiving more than eight doses ($n = 170$) showed 40% of patients free of disease, the group receiving 8 or fewer doses ($n = 78$) showed only 15% of cases of disease-free ($p < 0.0002$) [68].

In 2014, our group published the results of a small series of 15 patients treated with eight weekly doses of recirculating neoadjuvant MMC achieving a 66.6% CR and 33% PR. As in the previous case, the beneficial effect of CHT remained in time and, after 3 years of follow-up, disease-free survival was 85%, and only two recurrent patients were treated with TUR-B and intravesical adjuvant MMC [84].

The most comprehensive and recent neoadjuvant study was published by Lüdecke et al. [85]; the study group consisted of 271 patients treated with 8 weekly doses of neoadjuvant CHT with MMC (40 + 40 mg). After TUR-B they observed that 76.1% had CR and another 7.6% showed PR.

Unlike our study, all patients with CR were given consolidation adjuvant CHT (six doses every 6 weeks of MMC (20 + 20 mg) for a total of 9 months of treatment [73]. With this treatment, they observed that 80.6% of patients were free of recurrence at 2 years.

It is important to mention that this group included 59.8% of patients who had failed after BCG, but even there, the percentage of patients free of recurrence in this group was 41.7 and 66.7%, respectively, among those who were already resistant to BCG and those who had relapsed early after such treatment.

A comparative study of the recurrence rate after neoadjuvant CHT vs a meta-analysis with BCG shows that after 5 years of follow the CHT group showed 64% of patients free of disease compared to 22% expected in the BCG group ($p < 0.0001$) [86].

3.4. CHT adverse events

Most published works show that the side effects were higher with CHT than with standard MMC, but this difference was not statistically significant; furthermore, these effects were usually mild and reversible. CHT has less systemic effects and bladder retraction than BCG but has more local effects such as spasm, hematuria, and dysuria [71]. In some cases there were severe or permanent side effects such as urethral perforation or bladder retraction [4, 69, 70].

With the microwave technology, the most common adverse events during treatment were spasms of the bladder (21.6%) and bladder pain (17.5%). Bladder spasms tend to occur more frequently with neoadjuvant treatment (17.8 vs 10.7%; $p = 0.398$) [1]. Similar results were seen with BWT™ [70, 73] and Combat™ [69, 84] recirculant systems. Side effects are frequent, but almost all cases were grades 1 and 2.

In our experience, with almost 800 recirculant instillations, only 3.1% of doses were delayed, and less than 1% were not performed. The main reasons for delating were infection, hematuria, and irritative chemical cystitis. The only reasons for anticipated end of the treatment were allergy and intolerance to catheterization.

Approximately 6% of doses were interrupted before 60 min usually because of bladder spasms or pelvic discomfort [69, 84]. Those patients who didn't tolerate the first dose well were orally premedicated with 600 mgs of ibuprofen or antispasmodic treatment depending on if they had complained of pain or spasms. In selected cases, spasmolytic IV was administered during treatment. Both oral medications such as IV proved effective to achieve a good tolerance in subsequent doses of CHT.

3.5. Comparison of treatments assisted by devices

Those forms of intravesical chemotherapy in which any device is used to improve the efficacy of intravesical chemotherapy are called "device assisted." There are fundamentally two: Electromotive drug administration (EMDA) enhances the absorption of MMC by using iontophoresis. On the other hand, there is CHT which is based on heating the bladder with the instilled chemotherapeutic drug.

EMDA is based on creating an electric current through three physicochemical principles (*iontophoresis, electroosmosis, and electroporation*) able to increase the migration of an electrically charged molecule through the bladder wall molecule. In this chapter, we are not going to evaluate EMDA, but we recommend further investigation reading about it because it is a very interesting way to improve the effectiveness of intravesical chemotherapy.

EMDA has demonstrated reduction on tumoral recurrences compared to standard MMC. Some readers may want to know which delivery system is better, CHT or EMDA. Until now, there is no answer to this question; Colombo et al. [87] published in 2001 a pilot study with marker lesion which resulted in favorable results for CHT.

3.5.1. Microwave technology

The first CHT system approved for humans use was the Synergo™ system. It is a computer-embedded intravesical irrigation system combined with an energy-delivering unit. The system includes an RF generator that delivers radio-frequency energy at 915 MHz, a drug circulating unit, and a microprocessor with application-specific software. A triple lumen transurethral Foley catheter is used for drug intravesical instillation. It has thermocouples for bladder wall temperature monitoring and an RF antenna that radiates the bladder walls, causing phenotypical changes specifically in cancerous cells, creates membrane "micro-poring" and metabolic changes in these cells to increase the uptake of the drug, and enhances drug mobility (*becomes an active diffusion*). To avoid damaging temperatures being reached in the bladder, the Synergo™ system has a cooling circuit that keeps the intravesical temperature at acceptable levels.

Synergo™ system has been used for 15 years and has conclusive studies in both neoadjuvant and adjuvant settings. Clinical efficacy in high-risk patients (including BCG failures and CIS) has been proven. In fact, a 60% reduction of tumoral recurrences were observed when comparing to standard MMC has been demonstrated. Moreover, its superior results were maintained over periods of time as long as 10 years.

Both basic and clinical studies have shown a range of 4°C between different areas of the bladder when treated with Synergo™ [88]. This irregular distribution of the heat may be a significant inconvenience because it produces undertreated areas (40°C) or "cold spots," and others which were clearly cytotoxic temperatures are reached or "hot spots." In fact, the tip of the emitter rests at the posterior bladder wall producing burns in up to 60% of the patients which is not a serious problem that usually heals without complications

Another drawback, associated with its urethral catheter, which is 20fr, is that the microwave emitter is inside the probe which makes it very rigid, which makes it difficult to place for the clinician and uncomfortable for the patient. It may even cause urethral lesions in any of the repeated catheterizations required in a complete treatment. Kiss et al. [89], described that in a group of 21 patients treated with this device, 38% of them had to abandon the therapy because of the severity of the side effects including a case of urethral perforation.

The final drawback of the Synergo™ system is economical. As it is based on microwave technology, each disposable transurethral probe contains an expensive emisor—inside making the cost per patient quite high.

3.5.2. Heated recirculating fluid technology

An alternative way to apply heat to the bladder is those systems based on recirculation of a solution of chemotherapeutic drugs heated externally and reintroduced to the bladder through a three-lumen catheter. Two different devices using this technology are currently available, Combat HIVEC™ BRS and BWT™ systems which are based on simple technology and use inexpensive disposables that make it attractive for performing CHT in a sustainable public healthcare system.

Both use a three-lumen-modified Foley catheter (HIVEC™ 16fr and BWT™ 18fr) which is soft and flexible, avoiding most problems related to urethral catheterization compared to other technologies.

Both try to maintain the chemotherapeutic solution at a fixed temperature, but there are some differences between them.

The Combat HIVEC™ BRS system uses an external aluminum heat exchanger ensuring efficient heat transfer and accurate temperature control of 43°C within ±0.5°C should this be 0.5 of the set temperature in the inner urothelium while providing homogeneous drug distribution throughout the bladder. Because of the efficiency of its aluminum heat exchanger, it only needs 30 mL to prime the disposable set minimizing dilution and means that the chemotherapy only needs to circulate around the closed circuit at 200 mL/min to maintain the temperature accurately, and this minimizes the pressure exerted on the bladder. It has a range of safety controls, over temperature and high pressure, and auto cutoff function.

BWT™ uses external heating plates with plastic heat exchanger which delivers an exit temperature of 46.5°C to achieve an inlet temperature of 44.5°C of the chemotherapy fluid in order to maintain a temperature within ±2°C.

BWT™ disposable set has a priming volume greater than 50 mL, which increases dilution of the chemotherapy. It recirculates the chemotherapy at 300 mL/min in order to maintain temperature within 2°C, which creates more pressure in the bladder compared to Combat HIVEC™ BRS system.

Patient safety and comfort are paramount to Combat HIVEC™ BRS. To achieve it, some special characteristics have been added. Whenever is desired, progressive increase of heat up to the final temperature (5 min) can be employed, which increases tolerance in sensitive patients. Moreover, if the tip of the catheter is blocked by bladder mucosa or for any other reason, the system can reverse the direction of circulation resolving the problem, which in some cases could cause pain or device malfunction.

Some doubts have been raised whether recirculating systems can achieve effective transfer of heat into the bladder and if they are able to stable temperatures throughout the bladder wall. This question has been answered by Longo from Duke University (USA) [90]. Measuring temperature with 16 surgically placed submillimeter fiber-optic microprobes and silicone germanium thermistors in swines' pelvic organs and at different depths of the bladder wall as well as high-powered infrared cameras, they found a temperature gradient across the bladder wall (from urothelium to serosa) that was between 1.5 and 2°C, achieving a temperature across the inner urothelium of 42.9°C ±0.4.

Due to both devices being in use for very few years, the greatest drawback of recirculative systems is their limited number of studies and treated patients to confirm their effectiveness. To achieve it, Combat Medical Ltd. is performing multicentric studies in the UK and Spain, *across 20 hospitals*, called HIVEC™-I (303 patients), HIVEC™-II (259 patients), HIVEC™-R (68 patients), HIVEC™-PREMITO (151 patients), and HIVEC™-HR (50 patients), which are all recruiting and progressing well and should complete in 2017 with a complete population over 830 patients. Unfortunately, we have no information about ongoing studies performed with the BWT™ device. The main differences between all three devices may be seen in **Table 2**.

Device	**Synergo™**	**BWT™ system**	**Combat™**
Heat source	Intravesical 915 MHz microwave antenna *(Recirculating cooling system)*	External heating plates *(Recirculating heating system)*	External flat, low-volume heat exchanger *(Recirculating heating system)*
Target temperature and fluctuation	42.5 ± 3°C	44.5 ± 2°C	43 ± 0.5°C
Priming volume	±25 mL	±50 mL	±30 mL
Catheter characteristics	20fr Rigid (Radio-frequency emitter + cooling system inside)	18fr Flexible	16fr Flexible
Advantages	Strong supporting evidence *(neoadjuvant and adjuvant)* Long-term follow-up Proven superior to BCG Proven effectiveness against CIS Minimal dilution of MMC	Simple and cheap	Accurate temperature control and delivery Minimal dilution of MMC Good safety controls Proven effectiveness in sequential and neoadjuvant with medium-term follow-up Simple and easy to use Cheap
Disadvantages	Higher side effects Lower patient tolerance Intravesical hot and cold spots Expensive device and disposables Continuous operator control required throughout treatment	Limited clinical evidence Higher flow rates and operating pressure *(increase hematuria and reduce patient tolerance)* No pressure control or safety alarms	Limited evidence *(multicentric studies ongoing)*

Table 2. Characteristic of devices for intravesical CHT treatment.

3.6. Pharmacoeconomic evaluation

Bladder cancer is the most expensive tumor for public health services from the time of diagnosis to the patient's death [91].

We have studied the relationship between cost-effectiveness and budget impact of a neoadjuvant CHT in NMIBC patients and compared the results with standard treatment of BCG applying recurrence and progression values based on internationally accepted risk charts [92, 93].

For this reason, a model was designed from the perspective of a public health system after a follow-up of 3 years to compare the costs of implementing neoadjuvant CHT (*eight weekly instillations of 80 mg mitomycin C recirculating 43°C for 1 hour prior to TUR-B*) to costs of treating 15 patients with the same risk profile with standard adjuvant BCG treatment (*control group*). The actual costs related to available drugs, disposables, TUR-B, cold biopsy, and risk of tumor recurrence were included. Discarded model costs and follow-up diagnostic tests don't vary between the groups [94].

The model was built using information from actual study data, and estimated costs establish a favorable environment for neoadjuvant CHT in terms of cost to 3 years with a global minimum savings of 10.300 and 687 € per patient difference, all with improved effectiveness in the treatment. In fact, of the 15 patients pretreated with chemohyperthermia (*11 high risk and 4 medium risk*), the expected number of recurrences was reduced from 8 to 2 and progressions from 3 to 0. The conclusion of this study of 3 years is that neoadjuvant CHT is a cost-effective therapeutic strategy [94].

4. Take-home messages

4.1. Oncological results

Randomized studies have shown that CHT get the same or even better results than BCG in high-risk patients (T1GIII) regarding the free disease time, although its effectiveness in CIS has to be confirmed as well as tumoral progression

CHT reduced tumor recurrence by 60% compared to standard MMC in patients with intermediate-high-risk MMC and that these differences are maintained even years after treatment. Lower rates of progression vs standard MMC were also achieved but without significant differences.

Neoadjuvant CHT achieves tumoral eradication in two-third of intermediate-high-risk patients, and four-fifth are disease-free after 3 years of follow-up.

4.2. Tolerance

CHT has a nonsignificant higher side effects rate than standard MMC, but these are always low grade and transient. CHT has less systemic effects and bladder retraction than BCG but has more local effects such as spasm, hematuria, and dysuria.

4.3. Economics

Neoadjuvant CHT is a cost-effective therapeutic strategy against BCG treatment.

4.4. Indications

CHT is an undeniable option in BCG refractory tumors; those who are intolerant to BCG are unsuitable for radical cystectomy or in the context of an international BCG shortage.

Its use instead of MMC, both in adjuvant or neoadjuvant protocols, is promising options pending further evaluation.

Finally, the main pros and cons of CHT are condensed in **Table 3**.

Favorable arguments about its use	Contrary arguments about its use
- Improves results of standard MMC by 60% ($p < 0.001$) - Improvements in disease-free survival persist after 10 years vs standard MMC ($p < 0.002$) and 2 years vs BCG ($p < 0.008$) - Less systemic effects and bladder retraction than BCG - Bladder preservation rate to 10 years of 86 vs 79% CHT MMC cold (p = ns) - Useful in CIS and high-grade tumors - Excellent alternative to current or future shortage of BCG - Effective in BCG failures (41–66%) - As effective as BCG in CIS and T1G3 (89.5 vs 85.7%) - Lower rates of progression vs BCG (1.7 vs 2.8%, p = ns) - Reduces the overall cost of bladder cancer treatment (p = ns)	- The need for greater scientific evidence - Increased side effects vs normothermic MMC - Increases initial cost of adjuvant treatment - Operational problems by having a patient on a gurney for 60 min while medication is instilled instead of sending the patient home

Table 3. Pros and cons about chemohyperthermia.

Author details

Sousa-Escandón Manuel Alejandro*, Flores Carbajal Javier , Sousa-González Daniel and Rodriguez Gómez Silvia

*Address all correspondence to: sousa-alejandro@hotmail.com

Comarcal Hospital of Monforte, Monforte-Lugo, Spain

References

[1] Burger M, Catto J, Dalbagni G, Grossman H, Herr H, Karakiewicz P, et al. Epidemiology and risk factors of urothelial BC. Eur Urol, 63(2): 234–241, 2013

[2] Tomaszewski J, Smaldone M. Emerging intravesical therapies for management of NMIBC. Open Access J Urol, 2: 67–84, 2010.

[3] J Meyer, R Persad, D Gillatt. Use of bacille Calmette-Guérin in superficial bladder cancer. Postgrad Med J, 78(922): 449–454, 2002

[4] Lammers RJ, Witjes JA, Inman BA Leibovitch I, Laufer M, Nativ O, Colomo R. The role of a combined regimen with intravesical chemotherapy and hyperthermia in the management of non-muscle-invasive bladder cancer: a systematic review. Eur Urol, 60(1): 81–93, 2011.

[5] Madineh SM. Avicenna's canon of medicine and modern urology. Part III: other bladder diseases. Urol J, 6(2): 138–144, 2009

[6] Walton RJ, Sinclair WK. Radioactive solutions in the treatment of carcinoma of the bladder. Br Med Bull, 1(4096): 159–162, 1952

[7] Jones H, Swinney J. Thiotepa in the treatment of tumors of the bladder. The Lancet (British Ed.), 2(7203): 615–619, 1961

[8] Wataki S, Harada Y, Uzu K, et al. The identity of porfiromycin and methyl mitomycin. Antibiot Chemother (Northfield), 12: 469–471, 1962

[9] Ogawa H. Intracavitary treatment of tumors of the bladder with cytotoxic agent (mitomycin C) and radioactive phosphorus (32P). Nihon Hinyokika Gakkai Zasshi, 60(8): 717–723, 1969

[10] Shida K, Shimasaki J, Takahashi H, et al. Therapy and prognosis of bladder tumors–result of injection of mitomycin C into the bladder. Gan No Rinsho, 16(7): 737–744, 1970

[11] Kaufman JJ, Walther PJ, Smith RB, Skinner DG. Intracavitary mitomycin-C in the treatment of superficial urothelial tumors: a preliminary report. Trans Am Assoc Genitourin Surg, 71: 6–7, 1979

[12] Morales A, Eidinger D, Bruce AW. Intracavitary Bacillus Calmette-Guerin in the treatment of superficial bladder tumors. J Urol, 116(2): 180–183, 1976

[13] Bentley P. The vertebrate urinary bladder: osmoregulatory and other uses. Yale J Biol Med, 52: 563–568, 1979

[14] Soler R, Bruschini H, Martins JR, et al. Urinary glycosaminoglycans as biomarker for urothelial injury: is it possible to discriminate damage from recovery? Urology, 72(4): 937–942, 2008

[15] Mathai JC, Zhou EH, Yu W, et al. Hypercompliant apical membranes of bladder umbrella cells. Biophys J, 107(6): 1273–1279, 2014

[16] Alroy J, Weinstein RS. Intraepithelial asymmetric-unit-membrane plaques in mammalian urinary bladder. Anat Rec, 197(1): 75–83, 1980

[17] Flüchter SH, Hlobil H, Harzmann R, et al. Blood and tissue levels of mitomycin C after intravesical instillation. Urol Int, 38(6): 321–328, 1983

[18] Dalton JT, Wientjes MG, Badalament RA, et al. Pharmacokinetics of intravesical mitomycin C in superficial bladder cancer patients. Cancer Res, 51(19): 5144–5152, 1991

[19] Maffezzini M, Campodonico F, Manuputty E, et al. Systemic absorption and pharmacokinetics of single-dose early intravesical mitomycin C after transurethral resection of NMIBC. Urology, 82(2): 400–404, 2013

[20] M. Babjuk, W. Oosterlinck, R. Sylvester, et al. EAU guidelines on non-muscle-invasive urothelial carcinoma of the bladder, the 2011 update. Actas Urol Esp, 36: 389–402, 2012.

[21] Husillos A, Rodríguez E, Herranz Amo F, et al. The need for re-TUR of the bladder in non-muscle invasive bladder cancer: risk factors of tumor persistence in re-TUR specimens. Minerva Urol Nefrol, 66(4): 233–240, 2014.

[22] Divrik RT, Yildirim U, Zorlu F, Ozen H. The effect of repeat transurethral resection on recurrence and progression rates in patients with T1 tumors of the bladder who received intravesical mitomycin: a prospective, randomized clinical trial. J Urol, 175(5): 1641–1644. 2006

[23] Soloway MS, Masters S. Urothelial susceptibility to tumor cell implantation: influence of cauterization. Cancer, 46(5): 1158–1163, 1980

[24] Iborra JI, Ricos JV, Monrós JL, Dumont R, Casanova J, Solsona E. Results of a randomized, double blind prospective study of intravesical chemoprophylaxis with 2 drugs: adriamycin and mitomycin; and 2 ways of initiating the instillations: early and late. Effect on recurrence and progression. Arch Esp Urol, 45(10): 1001–1007, 1992

[25] Solsona E, Iborra I, Ricós JV, Monrós JL, Casanova J, Dumont R. Effectiveness of a single immediate MMC instillation in patients with low risk superficial bladder cancer: short and long-term follow-up. J Urol, 161(4): 1120–1123, 1999.

[26] Jung S, Chang H, Park C, et al. Effectiveness of an immediate Mitomycin C instillation in patients with superficial bladder cancer receiving periodic Mitomycin C instillation. Korean J Urol, 52(5): 323, 2011

[27] El-Ghobashy S, El-Leithy TR, Roshdy MM, El-Ganzoury HM. Effectiveness of a single immediate MMC instillation in patients with low risk NMIBC: short and long-term follow-up. J Egypt Natl Canc Inst, 19(2): 121–126, 2007

[28] Abern MR, Owusu RA, Anderson MR, et al. Perioperative intravesical chemotherapy in non-muscle-invasive bladder cancer: a systematic review and meta-analysis. J Natl Compr Canc Netw, 11(4): 477–484, 2013.

[29] Elmamoun M, Christmas T, Woodhouse C. Destruction of the bladder by single dose Mitomycin C for low-stage transitional cell carcinoma (TCC)–avoidance, recognition, management and consent. BJU Int, 113: 34–38, 2014

[30] Takahashi T, Habuchi T, Kakehi Y, et al. Clonal and chronological genetic analysis of multifocal cancers of the bladder and upper urinary tract. Cancer Res, 58(24): 5835–5841, 1998.

[31] Solsona E, Iborra I, Ricos JV, Monros JL, Rubio J, Almenar S. Clinical panurothelial disease in patients with superficial bladder tumors: therapeutic implications. J Urol, 167(5): 2007–2011, 2002.

[32] Turki O. Al Hussain MD, Akhtar M. Molecular basis of urinary bladder cancer. Adv Anat Pathol, 20: 53–60, 2013.

[33] Shelley MD, Court JB, Kynaston H, et al. Intravesical BCG versus MMC for Ta and T1 bladder cancer. Cochrane Database Syst Rev, (3): CD003231, 2003. PMID: 12917955 DOI: 10.1002/14651858.CD003231

[34] Malmstrom PU, Sylvester RJ, Crawford DE, et al. An individual patient data meta-analysis of the long-term outcome of randomised studies comparing intravesical mitomycin C versus Bacillus Calmette-Guerin for non-muscle-invasive bladder cancer. Eur Urol, 56(2): 247–256, 2009

[35] van der Zee J. Heating the patient: a promising approach? Annals Oncol, 13(8): 1173–1184, 2002

[36] Hildebrandt B, Wust P, Ahlers O, et al. The cellular and molecular basis of hyperthermia. Crit Rev Oncol Hematol, 43(1): 33–56, 2002

[37] Coley WB. The treatment of Inoperable Sarcoma by bacterial toxins (the mixed toxins of the streptococcus erysipelas and the Bacillus prodigiosus). Proc R Soc Med, 3: 1–48, 1910.

[38] Wust P, Hildebrandt B, Sreenivasa G, et al. Hyperthermia in combined treatment of cancer. Lancet Oncol, 3(8): 487–497, 2002

[39] Alexander HR. Isolation perfusion. In: DeVita VT Jr., Hellman S, Rosenberg SA, editors. *Cancer: Principles and Practice of Oncology*. Vol. 1 and 2. 6th ed. Philadelphia: Lippincott Williams and Wilkins, 2001.

[40] Falk MH, Issels RD. Hyperthermia in oncology. Internat J Hyperth, 17(1): 1–18, 2001

[41] Dewhirst MW, Gibbs FA Jr., Roemer RB, Samulski TV. Hyperthermia. In: Gunderson LL, Tepper JE, editors. *Clinical Radiation Oncology*. 1st ed. New York, NY: Churchill Livingstone, 2000.

[42] Kapp DS, Hahn GM, Carlson RW. Principles of hyperthermia. In: Bast RC Jr., Kufe DW, Pollock RE, et al., editors. *Cancer Medicine*. 5th ed. Hamilton, Ontario: B.C. Decker Inc., 2000.

[43] Feldman AL, Libutti SK, Pingpank JF, et al. Analysis of factors associated with outcome in patients with malignant peritoneal mesothelioma undergoing surgical debulking and intraperitoneal chemotherapy. J Clin Oncol, 21(24): 4560–4567, 2003

[44] Sessler DI. Thermoregulatory defense mechanisms. Crit Care Med, 37(7 Suppl): S203–S210, 2009.

[45] Rampersaud EN, Vujaskovic Z, and Inman BA. Hyperthermia as a treatment for bladder cancer. Oncology, 24(12): 1149–1155, 2010.

[46] Selawry OS, Goldstein MN, and Mc CT. Hyperthermia in tissue-cultured cells of malignant origin. Cancer Res, 17(8): 785–791, 1957.

[47] Coss RA, Dewey WC and Bamburg JR. Effects of hyperthermia on dividing Chinese hamster ovary cells and on microtubules in vitro. Cancer Res, 42(3): 1059–1071, 1982.

[48] Jäättelä M. Heat shock proteins as cellular lifeguards. Ann Med, 31(4): 261–271, 1999.

[49] Eppink B, Krawczyk PM, Stap J, and Kanaar R. Hyperthermia-induced DNA repair deficiency suggests novel therapeutic anti-cancer strategies, Int J Hyper, 28(6): 509–517, 2012.

[50] Dewey WC, Westra A, Miller HH, and Nagasawa H. Heat-induced lethality and chromosomal damage in synchronized Chinese hamster cells treated with 5-bromodeoxyuridine. Int J Rad Biol, 20(6): 505–520, 1971.

[51] Kluger MJ. The evolution and adaptive value of fever. Am Sci, 66(1): 38–43, 1978.

[52] Frey B, Weiss EM, Rubner Y, et al. Old and new facts about hyperthermia-induced modulations of the immune system. Int J Hyperth, 28(6): 28–42, 2012.

[53] Binder RJ and Srivastava PK. Peptides chaperoned by heat-shock proteins are a necessary and sufficient source of antigen in the cross-priming of CD8+ T cells. Nat Immunol, 6(6): 593–599, 2005.

[54] Srivastava P. Roles of heat-shock proteins in innate and adaptive immunity. Nat Rev Immunol, 2(3): 185–194, 2002.

[55] Srivastava P. Interaction of heat shock proteins with peptides and antigen presenting cells: chaperoning of the innate and adaptive immune responses. Ann Rev Immunol, (20): 395–425, 2002.

[56] Robins HI, Kutz M, Wiedemann GJ, et al. Cytokine induction by 41.8°C whole body hyperthermia. Cancer Lett, 97(2): 195–201, 1995.

[57] Chen Q, Fisher DT, Clancy KA, et al. Fever-range thermal stress promotes lymphocyte trafficking across high endothelial venules via an interleukin 6 trans-signaling mechanism. Nat Immunol, 12(7): 1299–1308, 2006.

[58] Dayanc BE, Beachy SH, Ostberg JR, and Repasky EA. Dissecting the role of hyperthermia in natural killer cell mediated anti-tumor responses. Int J Hyperth, 24(1): 41–56, 2008.

[59] Strauch ED, Fabian DF, Turner J, and Lefor AT. Combined hyperthermia and immunotherapy treatment of multiple pulmonary metastases in mice. Surg Oncol, 3(1): 45–52, 1994.

[60] Iwata K, Shakil A, Hur WJ, Makepeace CM, Griffin RJ, and Song CW, Tumour pO2 can be increased markedly by mild hyperthermia. Br J Cancer, 27(Suppl): S217–S221, 1996.

[61] Sun X, Xing L, Clifton Ling C, and Li GC. The effect of mild temperature hyperthermia on tumour hypoxia and blood perfusion: relevance for radiotherapy, vascular targeting and imaging. Int J Hyperth, 26(3): 224–231, 2010.

[62] Vaupel P, Kallinowski F, and Kluge M. Chapter "Pathophysiology of tumors in hyperthermia". In the book "Application of hyperthermia in the treatment of cancer", Vol. 107 of the series "Recent Results in Cancer Research": 65–75, Springer-Verlag Berlin – Heidelberg 1988.

[63] Haas GP, Klugo RC, Hetzel FW, et al. The synergistic effect of hyperthermia and chemotherapy on murine transitional cell carcinoma. J Urol, 132(4): 828–833, 1984

[64] Van der Heijden AG, Verhaegh G, Jansen CF, et al. Effect of hyperthermia on the cytotoxicity of 4 chemotherapeutic agents currently used for the treatment of transitional cell carcinoma of the bladder: an in vitro study. J Urol, 173(4): 1375–1380, 2005.

[65] Van der Heijden AG, Jansen CF, Verhaegh G, et al. The effect of hyperthermia on mitomycin-C induced cytotoxicity in four human bladder cancer cell lines. Eur Urol, 46(5): 670–674, 2004.

[66] Paroni R, Salonia A, Lev A, et al. Effect of local hyperthermia of the bladder on mitomycin C pharmacokinetics during intravesical chemotherapy for the treatment of superficial transitional cell carcinoma. Br J Clin Pharmacol, 52(3): 273–278, 2001

[67] Milla P, Fiorito C, Soria F, et al. Intravesical thermo-chemotherapy based on conductive heat: a first pharmacokinetic study with mitomycin C in superficial transitional cell carcinoma patients. Cancer Chemother Pharmacol, 73(3): 503–509. 2014

[68] Witjes A, Kees Hendricksen O, Grofit O, et al. Intravesical hyperthermia and MMC for carcinoma in situ of the urinary bladder: experience of the European Synergo working party. World J Urol, 27(3): 319–324, 2009

[69] Sousa A, Piñeiro I, Rodríguez S, Aparici V, Monserrat V, Neira P, et al. Recirculant hyperthermic IntraVEsical chemotherapy (HIVEC) in intermediate–high-risk non-muscle-invasive bladder cancer. Int. J. Hyperth, 32(4): 374–380, 2016

[70] Ekin RG, Akarken I, Zorlu F, Tarhan H, Kucuk U, Yildirim Z, Divrik RT. Intravesical bacillus Calmette-Guérin versus chemohyperthermia for high-risk non-muscle-invasive bladder cancer. Can Urol Assoc J, 9(5–6): 278–283, 2015.

[71] Arends T, Nativ O, Maffezzini M, Cobelli O, Canepa G, Verweij F, et al. Results of a randomized controlled trial comparing intravesical chemo-hyperthermia with mitomycin C versus BCG for adjuvant treatment of patients with intermediate and high risk NMIBC. Eur Urol, 69: 1046–1052, 2016

[72] Ekin RG, Akarken I, Cakmak O, Tarhan H, Celik O, Ilbey YO, et al. Results of intravesical chemo-hyperthermia in high-risk non-muscle invasive bladder cancer. Asian Pac J Cancer Prev, 16(8): 3241–3245, 2015.

[73] Colombo R, Salonia A, Leib Z, Pavone-Macaluso M, Engelstein D. Long-term outcomes of a randomized controlled trial comparing thermochemotherapy with mitomycin-C alone as adjuvant treatment for non-muscle-invasive bladder cancer (NMIBC). BJU Int, 107(6): 912–918; 2011

[74] Schrier B, Hollander M, van Rhijn B. Prognosis of muscle-invasive bladder cancer: difference between primary and progressive tumours and implications for therapy. Eur Urol, 45: 292–296, 2004

[75] Guzzo T, Magheli A, Bivalacqua T, et al. Pathological upstaging during radical cystectomy is associated with worse recurrence-free survival in patients with bacillus Calmette-Guerin-refractory bladder cancer, Urology 74(6): 1276–1280, 2009.

[76] Ayres B, Connor A, Corbishley C, Bailey M. 3-year single-centre UK experience of radiofrequency hyperthermia and mitomycin C in BCG failures. BJU Int, 106(Suppl s1), 2010

[77] Van der Heijden A., Kiemeney L, Gofrit O, et al. Preliminary European results of local microwave hyperthermia and chemotherapy treatment in intermediate or high risk superficial transitional cell carcinoma of the bladder. Eur Urol, 46: 65–72, 2004.

[78] Witjes J, Hendricksen K, Gofrit O, et al. Intravesical hyperthermia and mitomycin-C for carcinoma in situ of the urinary bladder: experience of the European Synergo working party. World J Urol, 27: 319–324, 2009

[79] Halachmi S, Moskovitz B, Maffezzini M, et al. Intravesical mitomycin C combined with hyperthermia for patients with T1G3 transitional cell carcinoma of the bladder. Urol Oncol, 29(3): 259–264, 2011

[80] Moskovitz B, Halachmi S, Moskovitz M, et al. 10-year single-center experience of combined intravesical chemohyperthermia for nonmuscle invasive bladder cancer. Future Oncol, 8(8): 1041–1049, 2012.

[81] Griffits TR. Secuential chemohyperthermia plus BCG in high risk NMIBC. Plenary session conference at the annual national congress of the Spanish Urological Association. Toledo-Spain. June 16, 2016.

[82] Colombo R, Da Pozzo LF, Lev A, et al. Local microwave hyperthermia and intravesical chemotherapy as bladder sparing treatment for select multifocal and unresectable superficial bladder tumors. J Urol, 159(3): 783–7, 1998.

[83] Colombo R, Rocchini L, Suardi N, et al. Neoadjuvant short-term intensive intravesical mitomycin C regimen compared with weekly schedule for low-grade recurrent non-muscle-invasive bladder cancer: preliminary results of a randomised phase 2 study. Eur Urol, 62(5): 797–802, 2012

[84] Sousa A, Inman B, Piñeiro I, et al. A clinical trial of neoadjuvant intravesical chemotherapy (HIVEC) for treating intermediate and high-risk NMIBC. Int J Hyperthermia, 30(3): 166–170, 2014

[85] Lüdecke G, Schäfer L, Nativ O, Witzsch U, Hanitzsch H, Hasner F, et al. Radiofrequence induced hyperthermia chemotherapy in high-risk NMIBC: Multiinstitutional, international outcome analysis of 271 treated patients with a follow-up time of more than 2 years. Eur Urol Suppl 14(2): e949–e949[a], 2015

[86] Di Stasi S, Riedl C, Verri C, et al. Is intravesical BCG alone still the only truly effective intravesical therapy for high risk non-muscle invasive bladder cancer? Poster 945 EAU congress Madrid, 2015

[87] Colombo R, Brausi M, Da Pozzo L, et al. Thermo-chemotherapy and electromotive drug administration of mitomycin C in superficial bladder cancer eradication. a pilot study on marker lesion. Eur Urol, 39(1): 95–100, 2001.

[88] Rath-Wolfson L, Moskovitz B, Dekel Y, Kugel V, Koren R. Combined intravesical hyperthermia and mitomycin chemotherapy: a preliminary in vivo study. Int J Exp Path, 84: 145–152, 2003

[89] Kiss B, Schneider S, Thalmann G, Roth B. Is thermochemotherapy with the synergo a viable treatment option in patients with recurrent non-muscle invasive bladder cancer?. Int J Urol 22: 158–162, 2015

[90] Longo T. Heat-targeted drug delivary using a novel conductive bladder hyperthermia device. International congress of hyperthermic oncology. New Orleans (USA): Duke University, April 11–15, 2016

[91] Botteman M, Pashos C, Redaelli A, Laskin B, Hauser R. The health economics of bladder cancer. Pharmacoeconomics, 21(18): 1315–1330, 2003

[92] Sylvester RJ, van der Meijden AP, Oosterlink W, et al. Predicting recurrence and progression in individual patients with stage Ta T1 bladder cancer using EORTC risk tables: a combined analysis of 2596 patients from seven EORTC trials. Eur Urol, 49(3): 466–477, 2006

[93] Fernandez-Gómez J, Madero R, Solsona E, Unda M, et al. Predicting nonmuscle invasive bladder cancer recurrence and progression in patients treated with bacillus Calmette-Guerin: the Cueto Scoring Model. J Urol, 182(5): 2195–203, 2009.

[94] Sousa A, Piñeiro I, Aparici V, Neira P, Monserrat V. Analysis of budgetary impact of non-muscle invasive bladder cancer of moderate-high risk by means of neoadjuvant hyperthermic chemotherapy compared to standard adjuvant treatment with BCG. Arh Esp Urol, 68(5): 482–492, 2015

Chapter 3

Cross-Polarization OCT for In Vivo Diagnostics and Prediction of Bladder Cancer

Elena Kiseleva, Gladkova Natalia, Streltzova Olga, Kirillin Mikhail, Maslennikova Anna, Dudenkova Varvara, Yunusova Katerina and Sergeeva Ekaterina

Additional information is available at the end of the chapter

http://dx.doi.org/10.5772/67473

Abstract

This chapter contains three parts covering recent efforts to increase the accuracy of optical coherence tomography (OCT) differential diagnostics of bladder pathologies. The first part compares the diagnostic efficacy of traditional OCT and cross-polarization OCT (CP OCT); CP OCT and fluorescence cystoscopy (FC) for detecting flat lesions in the bladder at the early stages of cancer. The second part contains a report on achievements in application of CP OCT for detection of recurrent carcinoma in the scar area that is a hardly distinguishable form of bladder cancer using an optimized CP OCT image analysis. The third part of the chapter reviews the results on CP OCT usage for in vivo diagnosis of the bladder cancer after radiation therapy of cervical cancer.

Keywords: cross-polarization optical coherence tomography (CP OCT), bladder cancer, collagen, laser scanning microscopy (LSM), radiation damage

1. Introduction

Bladder cancer can manifest in a variety of different forms, and chronic inflammation plays the key role in its development [1]. One of the origins of bladder cancer development is the side-effect of radiation therapy. The radiation therapy of the uterus or prostate cancer frequently induces substantial alterations in the bladder wall that may progress to bladder cancer. Such side-effects of the radiation therapy of pelvic organs are of particular interest, as they occur in the patients with predicted long life expectancy, and preservation of the life quality is of comparable importance with recurrence prevention [2]. In this situation, early detection of bladder cancer or pre-cancer manifestations, preferably non-invasive, is the key for timely treatment.

Traditionally, white-light cystoscopy is employed for detection of bladder cancer. Besides the invasiveness and potential risks, white light cystoscopy drawbacks include difficult detection of flat lesions, inaccurate tumor delineation, which leads to complete resection and inability to differentiate between inflammation and malignancy and to determine the tumor grade and stage. In clinical practice, the overcoming of these drawbacks strongly depends on the surgeon's experience [3].

In the last decade, the techniques for diagnosing bladder pathologies were complemented by optical coherence tomography (OCT) being actively introduced into clinical practice [4–6]. OCT is a modern optical non-invasive imaging technique based on the principles of reflectance low-coherence interferometry, which can provide a tissue image to the depths up to several millimeters with spatial resolution down to units of μm. Cross-polarization OCT (CP OCT) is an OCT modality where probing is performed by polarized light; and two conjugated images are being registered in the channels with polarization parallel and orthogonal to initial one (co- and cross-polarization channels, respectively).

Many OCT research groups develop their own approaches for differential diagnostic of early bladder cancer [3, 7, 8]. The combination of OCT diagnostics with image analysis and signal processing (e.g., histograms analysis [9, 10], extraction of optical properties [11], texture analysis [12, 13]) has a high potential for automated differential diagnostics. To bridge the gap between research and clinical use, the potential of CP OCT was systematically investigated for real-time and label-free imaging. Nowadays, the studies are focused on challenging problems such as hardly distinguishable forms of bladder disorders related with cancer. Alterations in normal tissue that occur in the early and late periods after radiation therapy are an actual problem of modern radiation oncology [14] where high potential of the CP OCT was demonstrated.

This chapter contains three parts covering recent efforts to increase the accuracy of OCT differential diagnostics of bladder pathologies. The first part compares the diagnostic efficacy of traditional OCT (equivalent to obtaining co-polarized image only), CP OCT (employing combination of cross-polarized and co-polarized images), and fluorescence cystoscopy (FC) for detecting flat lesions in the bladder at early stages of cancer. In the second part, we report on the recent achievements in application of CP OCT for detection of carcinoma recurrence in scar area using an optimized CP OCT image analysis/quantification platform. The platform is based on detecting alterations in the collagen compartment of interrogated tissue's extra-cellular matrix (ECM). The third part reviews the pilot results of CP OCT employment for in vivo evaluation of the severity of the bladder mucosa damage after radiation therapy of cervical cancer. In addition to morphological analysis with hematoxylin and eosin (H&E) and picrosirius red (PSR) staining, nonlinear laser scanning microscopy (LSM) study was performed to confirm the level of collagen damage and remodeling as a consequence of cancer invasion and radiation therapy.

CP OCT studies of human urinary bladder mucosa during in vivo endoscopic examination described in this chapter were performed with the "OCT 1300-U" system (IAP RAS, Nizhny

Novgorod, Russia). CP OCT device has a forward-looking (en-face) endoscopic probe with outer diameter 2.7 mm that is placed vertically to the mucous surface leaving an imprint on it, so the tissue is taken for histology from the same area and has the same orientation. The CP OCT system is based on superluminiscent diode with central wavelength 1300- and 100-nm bandwidth and has axial resolution ~15 μm and lateral resolution ~25 μm. Using the circular polarized probing light and two signal acquisition channels to detect scattered light that maintained initial polarization and change it to orthogonal one gave an advantage to assess co- ("co-polarized image") and cross-scattering ("cross-polarized image") properties of the tissue up to 1.8 mm in depth. CP OCT image size is 2.5 × 4.0 mm (width × height), image acquisition rate is 0.5 frames per sec. Refer to previous publications [15, 16] for more detailed system descriptions, including the optical phase retardation particulars to enable CP operation.

The fragments of the bladder mucosa from the sites of CP OCT inspection extracted in course of surgery and biopsy were subjects for further histological and LSM examination. Later, CP OCT images were compared to the morphological images. Histologic study included light microscopy with H&E staining and polarized light transmission microscopy with PSR staining for evaluation of structural and spatial organization of collagen fibers; LSM was applied in second harmonic generation (SHG) mode with excitation at the wavelength of 800 nm and spectral detection in the range of 362–415 nm to reveal the distribution of collagen fibers in the bladder mucosa.

The Ethics Committee of Nizhny Novgorod State Medical Academy for scientific research involving human subjects approved the clinical study. All patients voluntarily signed the informed consent for the study.

2. Efficacy of cross-polarization OCT in bladder cancer diagnosis: comparison with traditional OCT, fluorescence cystoscopy, and immunohistochemical study

The early OCT studies of bladder mucosa were performed with traditional time-domain modality equipped with an endoscopic probe. Diagnosis of early bladder cancer was the central topic of OCT studies in urology [4]. After 25 years, the OCT technique significantly improved resulting, in particular in cross-polarization time-domain OCT with common-path optical layout and two signal acquisition channels and in spectral CP OCT modification with the similar characteristics enabling 3D imaging.

2.1. Cross-polarization OCT and traditional OCT at bladder cancer

In course of introduction of CP OCT into clinical practice, the capabilities of this new technique for early bladder cancer detection were assessed in a comparative study with the traditional OCT. To assess the efficacy, the special test was developed. It consisted of two independent stages: assessing diagnostic capabilities of OCT (using a set of co-polarized images) for detecting neoplasia and assessing diagnostic capabilities of CP OCT (using a set of the same clinical cases, but with two images: in co- and in cross-polarization) for the same task. Statistical evaluation of the diagnostic efficacies of OCT and CP OCT was also performed independently. A total of 116 patients with localized flat suspicious lesions in the bladder were enrolled, 360 CP OCT images were acquired and analyzed. Statistical parameters and general results of the blind recognition tests of CP OCT and OCT images of flat suspicious lesions in the bladder are listed in Ref. [17].

Briefly, it was shown that CP OCT demonstrated higher sensitivity of 93.7% (vs. 81.2%, $p < 0.0001$), specificity 84% (vs. 70.0%, $p < 0.001$), and diagnostic accuracy 85.3% (vs. 71.5%, <0.001) in detecting early malignant changes in flat suspicious zones compared to the traditional OCT technique. The interobserver agreement index *kappa* increased from 0.68 to 0.82 when images in cross-polarization were added. The earlier analysis of more than 500 traditional OCT [4] and CP OCT images of benign and malignant states of the bladder [18] enabled us to formulate visual criteria for assessing CP OCT images in co- and in cross-polarization (**Table 1**).

Higher diagnostic efficacy of CP OCT in detecting early bladder cancer is associated with the ability to detect changes in epithelium and connective tissues. In previous works (see Refs. [17, 19]), it was demonstrated that OCT signal in cross-polarization (**Figure 1a**, upper image) is formed primarily due to cross-scattering from unaltered, well-organized type I collagen. This statement is based on the comparison of the signal level in cross-polarization with the brightness of PSR-stained collagen fiber luminescence in polarized light (**Figure 1j**).

It is known that collagen stained with PSR and examined with polarized light microscopy reveals its birefringent properties, visualized as bright pixels against the background of dark surrounding tissue elements (reference). Collagen type I has red and red-yellow color (thick fibers with thickness ~2–5 μm and higher) and collagen type III—green and green-white color (thin fibers with thickness ~1 μm). Red-orange color of thick-collagen fibers is also associated with densely packed collagen fibers indicative of their maturity [20].

CP OCT image characteristics		Benign processes in the bladder	Malignant processes in the bladder
In co-polarization:	OCT features	Sharp, high contrast between epithelium and connective tissue in more than 75% of the lateral range of image. The epithelial layer has lower signal level than the connective tissue layer	No or weak contrast between horizontal layers
	OCT type images	Benign	Cancer
In cross-polarization:	OCT features	Uniform signal that may have the structure of horizontal layers	No or weak signal, in some images in the form of isolated spots
	OCT type images	Benign	Cancer

Table 1. Visual criteria for assessing CP OCT images in co- and in cross-polarizations.

http://dx.doi.org/10.5772/67473

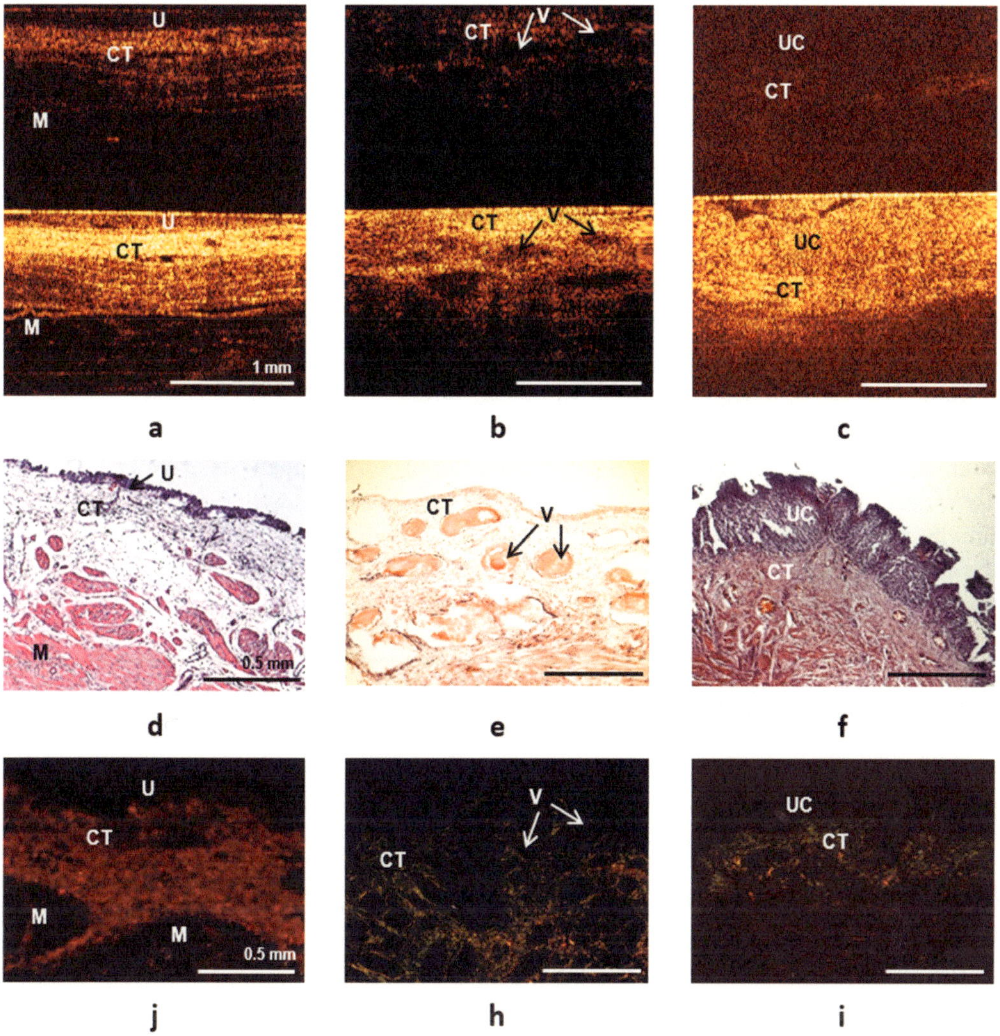

Figure 1. Bladder mucosa in normal state and in pathology. Normal (a, d, j), chronic exudative cystitis (b, e, h) and urothelial carcinoma Ia (c, f, i). CP OCT images (upper panel = cross-polarization, lower panel = co-polarization) (a, b, c), the corresponding histological slides stained with hematoxylin and eosin was used to confirm the diagnosis (d, e, f), stained with picrosirius red and examined with polarized light—to reveal the presence and type of collagen (j, h, i). U—urothelium, CT—connective tissue, M—muscle, V—vessel, UC—urothelial carcinoma.

The loss of collagen polarization properties due to its disorganization at neoplasia (**Figure 1f** and **i**) and massive inflammatory cellular infiltration significantly reduces OCT signal level in cross-polarization (**Figure 1c**, upper image). At the same time, CP OCT images at chronic cystitis in cross-polarization have regions with high-level signal (**Figure 1b**). It is caused by diffuse excessive synthesis and accumulation of collagen fibers (its assembly/bunching in the background of reduced degradation), especially around vessels (sclerosis of vessel wall; **Figure 1e** and **h**).

Based on the qualitative considerations above, it appears that morphological and polarization changes of collagen fibers properties in various pathological states are complex and interrelated.

2.2. Cross-polarization OCT, fluorescence cystoscopy, and immunohistochemical study at bladder cancer

Fluorescence cystoscopy (FC) is one of the techniques to search for regions suspicious for cancer on the inner bladder surface. However, it has low-positive predictive value [21, 22]. Immunohistochemical (IHC) markers for bladder cancer Ta-T2a have potential to improve the diagnostics and help in understanding of carcinogenesis at molecular level [23]. Unfortunately, this technique can be employed only ex vivo. Recent studies of years [19] were aimed to assess the diagnostic accuracy of the combined use of FC and CP OCT with quantitative estimation of OCT signal in cross-polarization for diagnosis of superficial bladder cancer in flat suspicious lesions and analyze epithelial and carcinoma cells proliferation activity by using IHC markers. A total of 26 patients with bladder cancer were enrolled in the study. Total amount of regions of interest was 92; 41 sites with urothelial carcinoma (28 cases of cancer in bladder tissue/13 cases of recurrent cancer in scar tissue) and 51 sites with inflammation (16 mild/35 severe).

The results of the study show that the combined use of FC and CP OCT with quantitative estimation of the OCT signal yields the diagnostic accuracy in detecting bladder cancer in flat suspicious zones of 93.6%, the sensitivity of 96.4%, specificity of 92.1%, positive predictive value of 87%, and negative predictive value of 97.9%, which indicates that the efficacy of this approach is close to that of biopsy.

Since chronic inflammation in the bladder is manifested by the increased proliferative activity of uroteliocytes, IHC study using cell proliferation markers (Ki-67, p53, and p63) allows for more accurate quantification of the urothelium state and the risk of developing urothelial neoplasm. Ki-67, p53, and p63 immunohistochemistry is suggested to be helpful to distinguish dysplastic changes and carcinoma in situ from reactive atypia. These IHC markers were applied for the study of areas where CP OCT images can be classified as cancer type.

The IHC study demonstrated a high level of p53 expression and high proliferation activity (the number of the cells positively stained for Ki-67, p53, and p63 exceeded 50%) in the regions of bladder cancer. Those indices were significantly higher ($p < 0.0001$) comparing to the regions with severe inflammation. In the regions with mild inflammation, the level of Ki-67, p53, and p63 did not differ significantly ($p > 0.05$) from those with severe inflammation [23]. This confirms that the increased urothelium proliferation level in patients with bladder cancer is typical for the entire mucosa and does not depend on the visual manifestations of the inflammatory process [1, 24].

The expression of p63 only in the areas of red fluorescence was significantly higher ($p = 0.038$) than in the areas without fluorescence. The expression of Ki-67 and p53 did not depend on fluorescence.

The study confirms enhanced expression of p53, p63, and Ki-67 in patients with recurrent, highly differentiated superficial (without invasion into the muscular layer) urothelial carcinoma with a low or moderate risk of disease progression [25–28].

Also, a correlation between CP OCT data and IHC markers data was demonstrated. High inverse correlation ($r = -0.732$; $r = -0.647$ and $r = -0.481$, respectively, $p < 0.002$) was demonstrated between the expression of p63, Ki-67, and p53 markers and the CP OCT signal in cross-polarization. The obtained correlations allow suggesting why signal in cross-polarization alters in cases of inflammation and neoplasia. Healthy tissue in co-polarization has a layered structure featuring the epithelium and connective stroma. A neoplastic process characterized by excessive proliferation of urothelial cells losing specificity is accompanied by activation of p53, p63, and Ki-67 expression. On the one hand, active proliferation can change optical properties of epithelial cells; on the other hand, it eventually leads to disorganization of collagen matrix. It was found that the higher the expression of the markers of cellular proliferation and adherence, the more intense loss of cross-scattering properties by connective tissue collagen is registered by CP OCT. However, it is still unclear which process is primary.

3. CP OCT for diagnostics of recurrent bladder cancer

Recurrent forms of bladder cancer are hard to distinguish by routine diagnostic approaches (cystoscopy). In the majority of cases, cancer recurrence at scar is hard to be distinguished from the scar tissue. In this situation, even OCT inspection may fail to provide adequate information due to visual similarity of scar and cancer in a diagnostic OCT image.

To develop an approach to distinguish the recurrence of bladder cancer and the scar, parallel in vivo CP OCT and morphological study of the level of cross scattering and state of collagen was performed for scar tissue (group 1, $n = 30$) and carcinoma in the scar area (group 2, $n = 28$). **Figure 2** shows that sometimes CP OCT images in the scar tissue (a) and in recurrence of carcinoma in scar area (d) look quite similar. In cross-polarization, the OCT signal is heterogeneous: in both cases, there are areas with high, reduced, or absence of signal (**Figure 2a** and **d**, upper images). Analysis of the structural organization of collagen fibers at fiber and tissue levels in the scar tissue (group 1) showed that in condition of chronic inflammation of the bladder mucosa areas of excessive synthesis and accumulation of collagen (see **Figure 2**, red and yellow color on PSR image (b) and intense green color on SGH image (c)) might alternate with not yet formed collagen fibers areas (see **Figure 2**, pale green color or dark areas on PSR image (b) and week or no SHG signal (c)). Analysis of the recurrence of carcinoma on a post-operation scar region (Group 2) revealed that on PSR image areas of carcinoma are dark, and collagen fibers are thin of pale-red color (**Figure 2e**); some of collagen fibers are destroyed. The collagen fibers are loosely stacked and surround cancer cells in SGH image (**Figure 2f**).

OCT image processing and quantification may give an additional valuable information for differentiation these two conditions. A number of previous studies demonstrate that the changes in polarization properties correlate with changes in collagen state [6, 23, 29–31] while

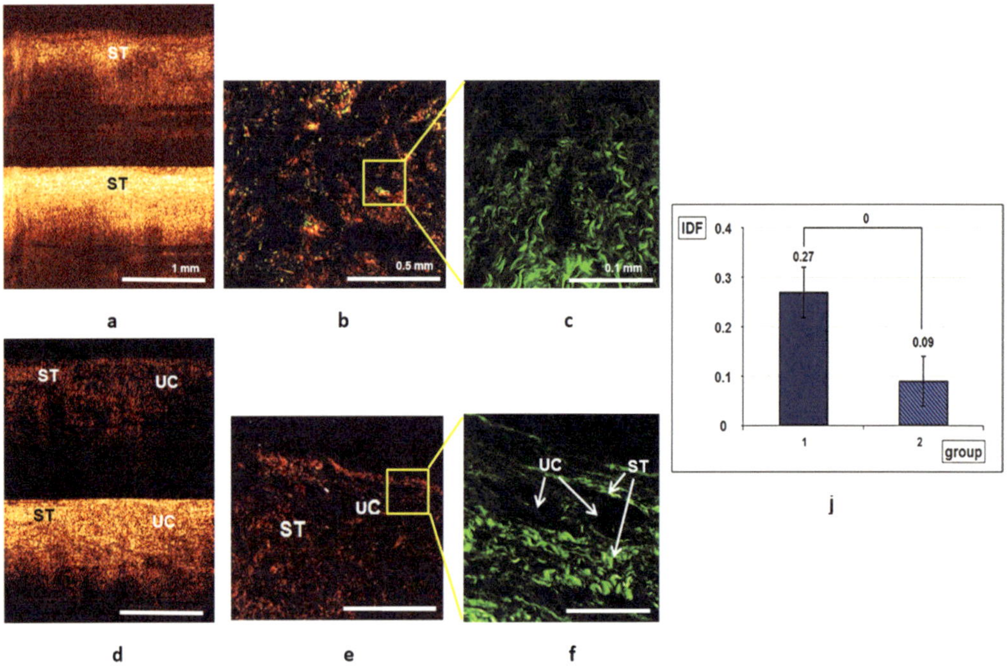

Figure 2. Scar tissue on the bladder mucosa and recurrence of urothelial carcinoma in the scar region. Group 1 (the upper row of images and left column on the diagram), Group 2—recurrence of carcinoma in the scar region (the lower row and left column on the diagram). CP OCT images (upper panel = orthogonal polarization, lower panel = initial polarization) (a, d); corresponding histological slides stained with picrosirius red and examined with polarized light (b, e); SHG images (c, f). ST—scar tissue, UC—urothelial carcinoma.

orientation and the degree of structural organization of collagen at fiber and tissue levels allowed to conclude on the presence of pathology [30]. Quantitative processing of CP OCT images was based on analysis of the cross-scattering properties of the bladder tissue [6]. An integral depolarization factor (IDF) was developed and successfully applied to quantify the collagen state within tissue [31]. IDF is defined as a ratio of the OCT signals in cross-polarization to co-polarization, both averaged over the transverse coordinates.

The results of comparing IDF in the groups of scar tissue (Group 1) and recurrence of urothelial carcinoma in the scar region (Group 2) are presented in **Figure 2j**. A statistically significant difference in IDF values between these two conditions is demonstrated ($p < 0.0001$), which testifies to the possibility of effective cystoscopic recognition of carcinoma in the region of post-operation scar with the IDF/CP OCT platform. It is known that collagen fibers are destroyed under the influence of tumor cell enzymes [32]; this likely decreased the resultant cross-polarization OCT signal. The quantitative assessment of CP OCT images obtained from the suspicious areas of postoperation scars can thus help in distinguishing the appearance of tumor in scar region.

Sensitivity, specificity, and diagnostic accuracy of separating recurrence of carcinoma in region of the bladder scar by quantitative assessment of CP OCT images with IDF are 93, 99, and 97%, respectively.

http://dx.doi.org/10.5772/67473

Intraoperative CP OCT monitoring of completeness of tumor removal was introduced into clinical practice (N.A. Semashko Nizhny Novgorod Regional Hospital) allowing minimizing the number of cancer recurrences at postoperative scar regions.

4. CP OCT for in vivo detection of bladder cancer after radiation therapy

The third paragraph of the chapter reviews the pilot results on CP OCT employment for in vivo detection of the bladder cancer after radiation therapy of cervical cancer.

Bladder cancer that occurs after radiation therapy of malignant neoplasms of the pelvic organs is a special problem in clinical urology. According to European Association of Urology, there is a two- to four-fold increase in the risk of secondary malignant tumors development in the bladder after radiotherapy of tumors of pelvic organs [33]. Recent studies [34, 35] confirmed the increase in the risk of bladder cancer for 1.5–4 times after the course of radiotherapy.

Alterations of normal bladder tissue occurring in the early and late periods after radiotherapy are an unsolved problem in modern radiation oncology [36]. The early side-effects include changes developed in the course of radiotherapy and 100 days after it. Radiation damages that appear after 3 months since radiotherapy procedure are treated as late; sometimes, they may occur in years after irradiation. In addition, in recent years, late effects resulting from long-term persistent severe acute radiation damage called "consequential late effects" are distinguished separately [37]. Specifically, late radiation-induced adverse events are of significant clinical importance [14]. Their severity can vary from clinically insignificant structural abnormalities to severe complications that have a great impact on the quality of patient's life (Cancer Therapy Evaluation Program) [38]. Different classifications including CTCAE, RTOG/EORTC, RILIT, and LENTSOMA were employed to determine the severity of post-radiation damage to normal tissues. Currently, the classification developed by Radiotherapy Oncology Group in collaboration with the European Organization for Research and Treatment of Cancer (RTOG/EORTC, 1995) is the most common classification scale for radiation complications (**Table 2**).

When bladder cancer appears in the irradiated and altered tissues, it becomes extremely difficult to diagnose cancer against edema, hemorrhage, and pronounced changes in the mucosa. Therefore, there is a challenge to differentiate changes induced by ionizing radiation and the changes caused by the tumor growth by standard clinical methods. In this situation, optical diagnostic techniques can play a crucial role in establishing the correct diagnosis.

In our clinical practice during last 2 years, a situation where CP OCT inspection allowed to diagnose bladder cancer in patients previously received radiotherapy for cervical cancer was met twice. Both patients have tumors developed at the background of severe (Grades 3 and 4) late side-effects of radiotherapy (**Table 2**).

Patient T., 65 years old, was hospitalized in urology department for vesico-urinary fistula. In January 2014, she was diagnosed with cervical cancer T3N0M0 (stage III). She received a concurrent chemoradiation therapy (external beam irradiation in a dose of 40 Gy, single dose

Organ tissue	Bladder
Grade 0	None
Grade 1	Slight epithelial atrophy, minor telangiectasia (microscopic hematuria)
Grade 2	Moderate frequency Generalized telangiectasia Intermittent macroscopic hematuria
Grade 3	Severe frequency and dysuria Severe generalized telangiectasia (often with petechiae) Frequent hematuria Reduction in bladder capacity (<150 cc)
Grade 4	Necrosis/contracted bladder (capacity <100 cc) Severe hemorrhagic cystitis
Grade 5	Death directly related to radiation late effects

Table 2. Classification of late radiation bladder damage (RTOG/EORTC, 1995).

2 Gy), brachytherapy in a dose of 25 Gy, single dose 5 Gy). In 18 months after radiation therapy, urine outflow from the vagina and blood in urine appeared. Ultrasound study revealed serozometra and right-side hydronephrosis. Laboratory blood tests showed signs of kidney failure. The right-side nephrostomy under ultrasound control and optical inspection of the bladder was made in November 2015. Cystoscopy revealed an organized blood clot within the bladder cavity. After bladder cavity dilatation, it was found that the bladder bottom was absent resulting in, a fistula defect of 3.5–4.0 cm in diameter. Bullous fabric with disintegration was revealed at the edge of the fistula. Mucosa of the bladder walls was hyperemic and hydropic (**Figure 3a**). Ureteral orifices were not visualized. Therefore, cystoscopy picture was consistent with the picture of Grade 4 radiation bladder damage (fistula, bleeding).

At the same time, bladder mucosa was studied with CP OCT; images of back left and right walls and around the fistula defect were acquired. CP OCT image of the back wall (**Figure 3c**) demonstrates the classic picture of chronic inflammation. Despite contrasted layers in co-polarization and high-level signal from connective tissue fibrosis in cross-polarization, both images feature edema (dark elongated areas, which have vertical shadows) and homogeneous areas originating from inflammatory cell infiltration of the stroma.

CP OCT image of the fistula edge (**Figure 3b**) manifests bullous features: in co-polarization, the image is mostly structureless: only the small area of image in the left has layers of epithelium (the first layer, may be with dysplastic changes), underlying connective tissue (the second layer, brighter) and below the signal abruptly falls (this area is suspicious to cancer); the central and the right side of the image are structureless, indicating neoplasia (**Figure 3b**). In cross-polarization, there is no pronounced signal, which approves the presence of neoplasia, and only small area in left side of the image corresponding to connective tissue demonstrates low-level signal. This flat zone is the suspicious area of the CP OCT image and transurethral biopsy was taken from this site. Morphologically, invasive

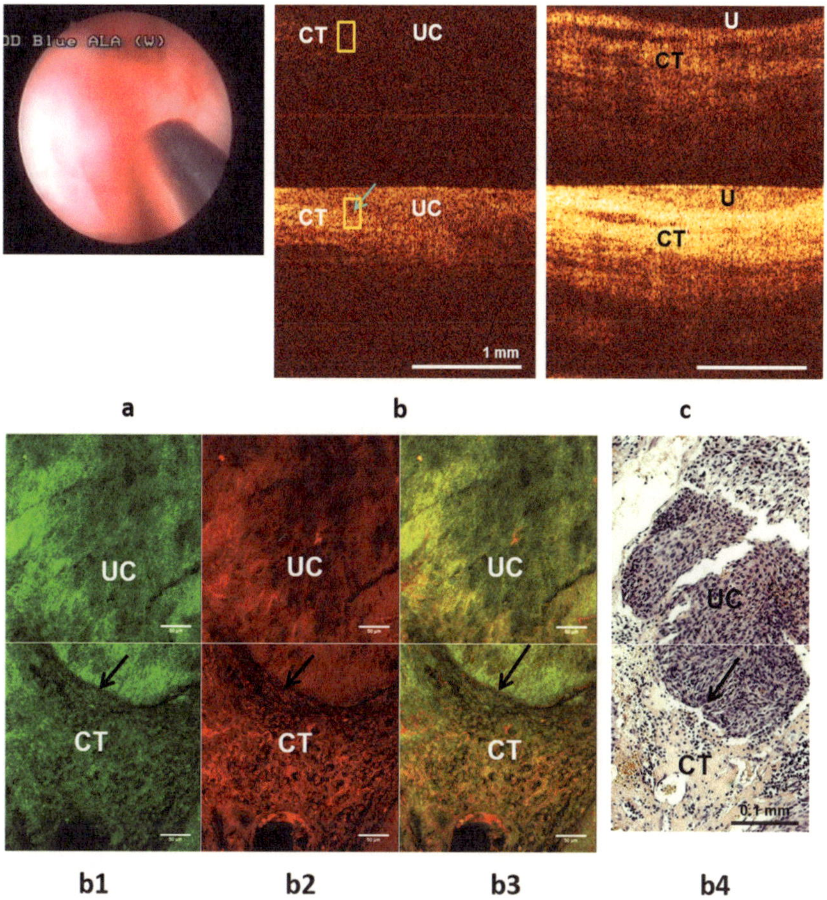

Figure 3. CP OCT guided biopsy of bladder mucosa and LSM study of extracellular matrix in 18 months after the end of radiation therapy. Cystoscopy image of the back wall in a moment of CP OCT study (a), CP OCT images (upper panel = cross-polarization, lower panel = co-polarization): image of tissue suspicious to cancer from border of fistula b), image of benign tissue from the back wall (c), LSM images (SHG (b1), 2PEF (b2) and combined SHG-2PEF (b3)) and histology (H&E) (b4) corresponding to CP OCT image (b). CT—connective tissue; U—urothelium; UC—urothelial carcinoma; arrows indicate border of carcinoma growth; yellow rectangle in (b) indicates area of LSM imaging (b1–b3).

transitional cell carcinoma Grade 2 was diagnosed (**Figure 3b4**). Conglomerates of cancer cells grow into the mucosa and submucosa layers of the bladder wall (area with low signal in co- and dark area in cross-polarization in **Figure 3b**, border of connective tissue is indicated with blue arrow). Carcinoma cells were localized deeper in connective tissue at the one side, whereas at the other side, it starts from the surface. Owing to CP OCT, biopsy was performed and urothelial carcinoma Grade 2 was detected while visually this area looked like inflammation.

We suppose that radiation induced damage of bladder connective tissue induced carcinoma development. In cross-polarization (left side of image), a low level signal from connective tissue is observed, originating from exudative inflammation process. Morphological analysis revealed congestion, swelling, lymphoid cell infiltrates in mucosa, and, important to mention, degenerative changes in collagen that cause decrease in cross-polarization OCT signal.

In order to determine more accurately the condition of collagen and elastic fibers in connective tissue of mucosa layer multiphoton, microscopy study was conducted. Confocal laser scanning microscope (LSM 710, Carl Zeiss, Germany) was used at the excitation wavelength of 800 nm. Detection was performed simultaneously in two channels by using filters in the wavelength ranges of 362–415 nm and 480–554 nm, with the aim to detect signals indicating SHG emission (green color in the images) and 2PEF emission (red color in the images), respectively. This approach allowed visualization of the collagen (seen in SHG) and primary elastin (seen in 2PEF) fibers in the walls of the bladder within the unstained, dewaxed sections with a thickness of 10 μm.

Two LSM images were combined to demonstrate the boundary between urothelial carcinoma and connective tissue (**Figure 3b1–b3**, the boundary is indicated with black arrow). Numerous small holes in the connective tissue corresponded to inflammatory infiltration, collagen is primary disorganized and looks homogeneous without clearly distinguished fibers (**Figure 3b1**), and elastic fibers are also damaged: they produced weak signal and are presented by fragments in a small amount (**Figure 3b2**). LSM study confirms that the connective tissue of the bladder after radiation therapy of pelvic organs has destructive changes that are preserved for the long time after treatment and in conjunction with chronic inflammation such condition can serve as a background for the cancer development.

Patient N., 41 years old, was urgently hospitalized in urology department with the diagnosis of chronic urinary retention. In 2014, she was diagnosed with cervical cancer T2bN0M0 (stage II), concurrent chemoradiation therapy (external beam irradiation in a dose of 40 Gy, brachytherapy in a dose of 25 Gy, single dose of 5 Gy) was held. In 20 months after the end of chemoradiotherapy, the patient became complaining of difficulty in urinating.

An ultrasound revealed pelvic adhesions, as well as the fact of bladder atony. Trocar cystostomy and cystoscopy study was done. Cystoscopically (**Figure 4a**), the mucous membrane of the bladder was shiny, whitish, trabecular, with tissue granulation on the back wall and in the triangle area; the bladder neck is loose, with a rough surface. Visually, three areas on mucosa were suspicious: in the center of the neck, in the neck close to the right wall, and close to the back wall. The CP OCT study of these areas was conducted, and then three biopsies were taken. Histology revealed presence of urothelial carcinoma Grade 3 complexes in two locations: in the center of the neck and in the neck close to the right wall (**Figure 4b4** and **c4**), where suspicious type of CP OCT images was obtained (**Figure 4b** and **c**). Both images have some features are not common for benign states. They contain structureless low signal areas without clear borders in co- and cross-polarizations at the lower part of the mucosa layer (first layer with a high level signal), and there is no epithelium layer usually manifested by middle intensity signal above the mucosa layer. Moreover, OCT signal from connective tissue in cross-polarization is homogeneous, whereas in norm and inflammation state, an image shows more or less distinct horizontally orientated structures.

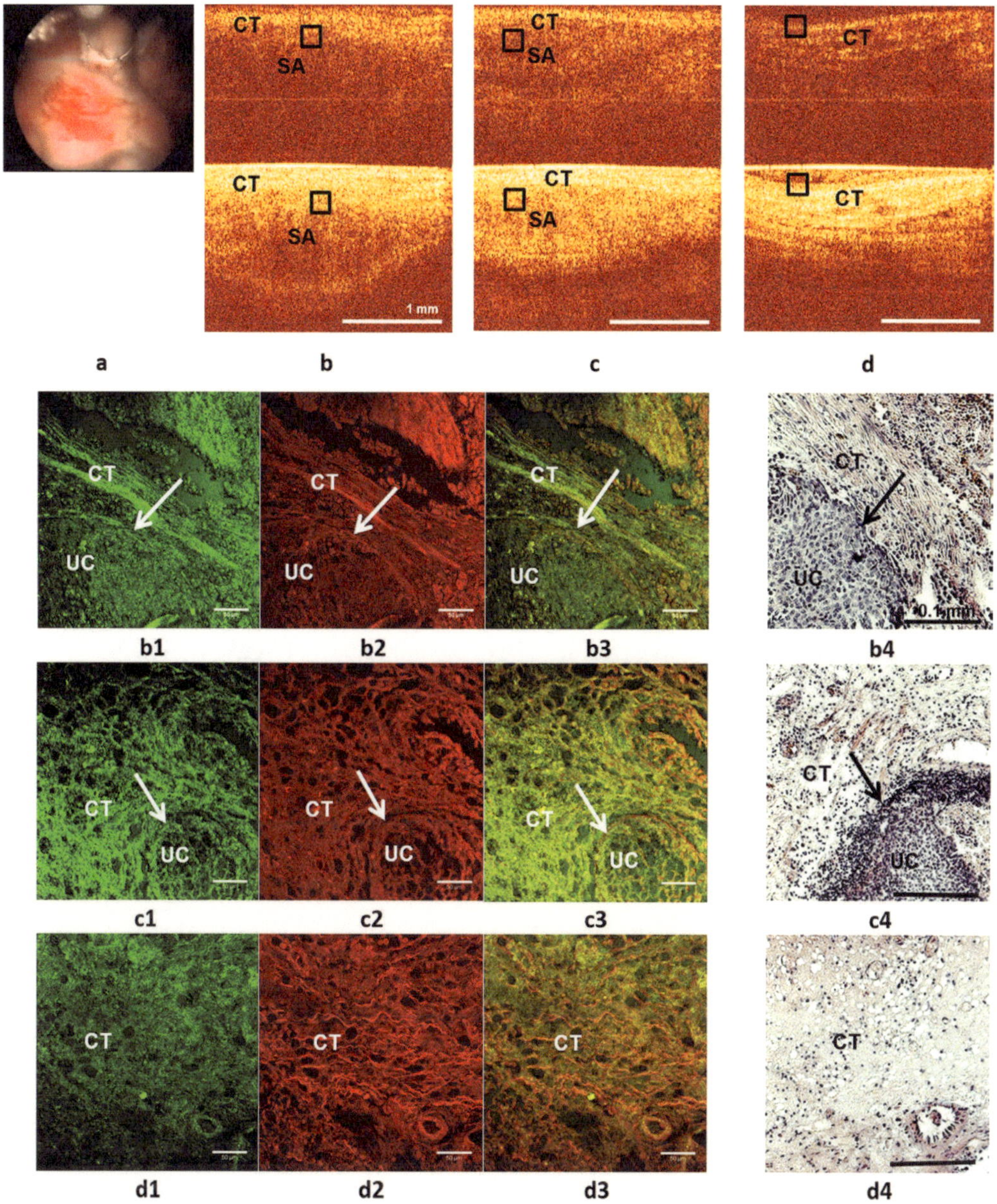

Figure 4. CP OCT of suspicious areas of bladder mucosa and LSM study of extracellular matrix in 20 months after the end of radiation therapy. Cystoscopy image of bladder neck with a loop of resectoscope at the time of biopsy (a), CP OCT images (upper panel = cross-polarization, lower panel = co-polarization): image of suspicious tissue at the bladder neck (b), image of suspicious tissue at the right wall close to the neck (c), image of bening tissue at the back wall (d), LSM images (SHG (b1, c1, d1), 2PEF (b2, c2, d2) and combined SHG-2PEF (b3, c3, d3)) and histology (H&E) (b4, c4, d4) corresponding to CP OCT images (b, c, d). CT—connective tissue; SA—suspicious area; UC—urothelial carcinoma; arrows indicate borders of carcinoma growth; black rectangle in (b, c, d) indicates area of LSM imaging (b1–b3, c1–c3, d1–d3, correspondingly).

CP OCT image of the third visually suspicious area (bladder neck close to the back wall) demonstrates the picture of chronic inflammation (**Figure 4d**) described above. Histology confirms supposed diagnosis: edemas, acute plethora, and round cells infiltration in the mucosa were present (**Figure 4d4**).

LSM images of bladder wall for the patient N. revealed that predominant amount of the fibers produces homogeneous signal similar to the previous case (**Figure 4c1–c3** and **d1–d3**). Only a few individual fibers of collagen and elastin are distinguished. This indicates disorganization processes in extracellular matrix. Loose network and holes in connective tissue in LSM images correspond to morphologically verified inflammation: edema and round a (**Figure 4c4** and **d4**).

Urothelial carcinoma in LSM images looks different: in the bladder neck, collagen in carcinoma is not organized (homogeneous SHG signal, **Figure 4b1**); however, close to the tumor, collagen fibers are straight, densely arranged, and have a prevailing orientation. This may point to aggressive and long-time growth of the carcinoma that starts to produce its own stroma and change the environment around to facilitate the invasion [32, 39]. In the neck close to the right wall, the carcinoma contains no elastic fibers and minimal amount of collagen organized in thin wavy fibers like in surrounding connective tissue, what may indicate infiltrative dissemination of carcinoma cells into loosely packed extracellular matrix **(Figure 4c1–c3**).

The described clinical cases show that extracellular matrix of bladder mucosa after radiation therapy of pelvic organs manifests dystrophic changes that could originate from the side-effects of radiation exposure and subsequent chronic inflammation. Rate of the bladder synchronic cancer in this case is up to 1.5–4 times larger as compared to nonirradiated bladder [34]. We suppose that disorganized collagen and elastic network in mucosa could also promote carcinoma fast growth and facilitate its invasion.

These examples demonstrate that to the patients, who undergone radiation therapy, a special attention and monitoring in the follow-up are required to prevent possible development of radiation induced urothelial carcinoma or detects it as early as possible. In this situation, CP OCT is an excellent minimally invasive tool for bladder mucosa inspection and evaluation of connective tissue state based on data in cross-polarization.

5. Conclusions

This chapter highlighted a novel diagnostic method, CP OCT, with high potential application for bladder pathology diagnosis. CP OCT can be considered an effective complementary in vivo technique to assess flat suspicious lesions in the bladder initially detected by white light or/and fluorescence cystoscopy, whereas the efficacy of these cystoscopy modalities alone or combined with traditional OCT is much lower.

Analysis and quantitative assessment of CP OCT images confirmed the presence of cross-scattering properties of connective tissue stroma in human mucosa that are determined by well-defined spatial and structural organization of collagen matrix. Collagen fibers undergo significant changes as a result of pathological processes which affect their cross-scattering properties that can be detected and quantified in vivo with CP OCT.

An approach to quantitative, robust, and potentially automated assessment of CP OCT images reflecting the state of bladder collagen fibers was developed. It was shown that IDF can be applied to in vivo detection of clinically relevant pathological states in urology. Differentiating between carcinoma recurrence at post-operation scar and tumor-free scar resulted in diagnostic accuracy of 97%. Thus, CP OCT and IDF quantification have promising potential to visualize and quantify the structural and spatial organization of CF in bladder tissues for clinical disease assessment including differential diagnosis applications.

Acknowledgements

This study was financially supported by the Russian Science Foundation, agreement no. 14-15-00538 (EBK, NDG, VVD) and the grants of the Russian Foundation for Basic Research No. 15-32-20250 (MYuK) and No. 16-07-00655 (OSS, AVM, KEYu).

Author details

Elena Kiseleva[1*], Gladkova Natalia[1], Streltzova Olga[1], Kirillin Mikhail[2], Maslennikova Anna[1], Dudenkova Varvara[1], Yunusova Katerina[1] and Sergeeva Ekaterina[2]

*Address all correspondence to: kiseleva84@gmail.com

1 Nizhny Novgorod State Medical Academy, Institute of Biomedical Technologies, Nizhny Novgorod, Russia

2 Institute of Applied Physics of the Russian Academy of Sciences, Nizhny Novgorod, Russia

References

[1] Gakis G. The role of inflammation in bladder cancer. Adv Exp Med Biol. 2014;**816**:183-196. DOI: 10.1007/978-3-0348-0837-8_8.

[2] Fiorino C., Valdagni R., Rancati T., Sanguineti, G. Dose-volume effects for normal tissues in external radiotherapy: pelvis. Radiother Oncol. 2009;**93**(2):153-167. DOI: 10.1016/j.radonc.2009.08.004.

[3] Liu J.J., Droller M.J., Liao J.C. New optical imaging technologies for bladder cancer: considerations and perspectives. J Urol. 2012;**188**(2):361-368. DOI: 10.1016/j.juro.2012.03.127.

[4] Zagaynova E., Gladkova N., Shakhova N., Gelikonov G., Gelikonov V., Zagaynova E. Endoscopic OCT with forward-looking probe: clinical studies in urology and gastroenterology. J Biophotonics. 2008;**1**(2):114-128. DOI: 10.1002/jbio.200710017.

[5] Lee C.S., Yoon C.Y., Witjes J.A. The past, present and future of cystoscopy: the fusion of cystoscopy and novel imaging technology. BJU Int. 2008;**102**(9 Pt B):1228-1233. DOI: 10.1111/j.1464-410X.2008.

[6] Kiseleva E.B., Kirillin M.Yu., Feldchtein F.I., Vitkin I.A., Sergeeva E.A., Zagaynova E.V., Streltzova O.S., Shakhov B.E., Gubarkova E.V., Gladkova N.D. Differential diagnosis of human bladder mucosa pathologies in vivo with cross-polarization optical coherence tomography. Biomed Opt Express. 2015;**6**(4):1464-1476. DOI: 10.1364/BOE.6.001464.

[7] Ren H., Yuan Z., Waltzer W., Shroyer K., Pan Y. Enhancing detection of bladder carcinoma in situ by 3-dimensional optical coherence tomography. J Urol. 2010;**184**(4):1499-1506. DOI: 10.1016/j.juro.2010.05.087.

[8] Ikeda M., Matsumoto K., Choi D., Nishi M., Fujita T., Ohbayashi K., Shimizu K., Iwamura M. The impact of real-time 3d imaging by ultra-high speed optical coherence tomography in urothelial carcinoma. BMC Urol. 2013;**13**(65). DOI: 10.1186/1471-2490-13-65.

[9] Kirillin M., Panteleeva O., Yunusova E., Donchenko E., Shakhova N. Criteria for pathology recognition in optical coherence tomography of fallopian tubes. J Biomed Opt. 2012;**17**(8):081413-081421. DOI: 10.1117/1.JBO.17.8.081413.

[10] Yang Y., Wang T., Biswal N.C., Wang X., Sanders M., Brewer M., Zhu Q. Optical scattering coefficient estimated by optical coherence tomography correlates with collagen content in ovarian tissue. J Biomed Opt. 2011;**16**(9):090504. DOI: 10.1117/1.3625247.

[11] Ejofodomi O. Measurement of optical scattering coefficient of the individual layers of the human urinary bladder using optical coherence tomography. ISRN Biomed Imaging. 2014;**2014**. 1-4. DOI: 10.1155/2014/591592.

[12] Kirillin M., Panteleeva O., Agrba P., Pasukhin M., Sergeeva E., Plankina E., Dudenkova V., Gubarkova E., Kiseleva E., Gladkova N., Shakhova N., Vitkin A. Towards advanced OCT clinical applications. In: Lilge L.D., Sroka R., editors. Medical Laser Applications and Laser-Tissue Interactions VII; July 15, 2015; Munich, Germany. Proc. SPIE; 2015. p. 9542. DOI: 10.1117/12.2183794.

[13] Lindenmaier A.A., Conroy L., Farhat G., DaCosta R.S., Flueraru C., Vitkin I.A. Texture analysis of optical coherence tomography speckle for characterizing biological tissues in vivo. Opt Lett. 2013;**38**(8):1280-1282. DOI: 10.1364/OL.38.001280.

[14] Dorr W. Pathogenesis and repair of normal tissue damage. Radiother Oncol. May 2011;**99**(Supp 1):S135. DOI: 10.1016/S0167-8140(11)70460-1.

[15] Gelikonov V.M., Gelikonov G.V. New approach to cross-polarized optical coherence tomography based on orthogonal arbitrarily polarized modes. Laser Phys Lett. 2006;**3**(9):445-451. DOI: 10.1002/lapl.200610030.

[16] Gubarkova E.V., Dudenkova V.V., Feldchtein F.I., Timofeeva L.B., Kiseleva E.B., Kuznetsov S.S., Shakhov B.E., Moiseev A.A., Gelikonov G.V., Vitkin A., Gladkova N.D. Multi-modal optical imaging characterization of athero-sclerotic plaques. J Biophotonics. 2016;**9**(10):1009-1020. DOI 10.1002/jbio.201500223.

[17] Gladkova N.D., Streltsova O.S., Zagaynova E.V., Kiseleva E.B., Gelikonov V.M., Gelikonov G.V., Karabut M.M., Yunusova K.E., Evdokimova O.V. Cross polarization optical coherence tomography for early bladder cancer detection: statistical study. J Biophotonics. 2011;**4**(7–8):519-532. DOI: 10.1002/jbio.201000088.

[18] Gladkova N.D., Zagaynova E.V., Streltsova O.S., Kiseleva E.B., Karabut M.M., Snopova L.B., Yunusova E.E., Tararova E., Gelikonov V.M. Advantages of cross-polarization endoscopic optical coherence tomography in diagnosis of bladder neoplasia. In: Kollias N., Choi B., Zeng H., Malek R.S., Wong B.J.F., Gregory K.W., Tearney G.J., Marcu L., Hirschberg H., Madsen S.J., Mandelis A., Mahadevan-Jansen A., Jansen E.D., editors. Photonic Therapeutics and Diagnostics VI; January 23, 2010; San Francisco, California. Proc SPIE; 2010. p. 754813. DOI: 10.1117/12.841810.

[19] Gladkova N., Kiseleva E., Robakidze N., Balalaeva I., Karabut M., Gubarkova E., Feldchtein F. Evaluation of oral mucosa collagen condition with cross-polarization optical coherence tomography. J Biophotonics. 2013;**6**(4):321-329. DOI: 10.1002/jbio.201200059.

[20] Lattouf R., Younes R., Lutomski D., Naaman N., Godeau G., Senni K., Changotade S. Picrosirius red staining: a useful tool to appraise collagen networks in normal and pathological tissues. J Histochem Cytochem. 2014;**62**(10):751-758. DOI: 10.1369/0022155414545787.

[21] Mowatt G., N'Dow J., Vale L., Nabi G., Boachie C., Cook J.A., Fraser C., Griffiths T.R. Photodynamic diagnosis of bladder cancer compared with white light cystoscopy: systematic review and meta-analysis. Int J Technol Assess Health Care. 2011;**27**:3-10. DOI: 1017/s0266462310001364.

[22] Elferink O.P., Witjes J.A. Blue-light cystoscopy in the evaluation of non-muscle-invasive bladder cancer. Ther Adv Urol. 2014;**6**(1):25-33. DOI: 10.1177/1756287213510590.

[23] Gladkova N., Kiseleva E., Streltsova O., Prodanets N., Snopova L., Karabut M., Gubarkova E., Zagaynova E. Combined use of fluorescence cystoscopy and cross-polarization OCT for diagnosis of bladder cancer and correlation with immunohistochemical markers. J Biophotonics. 2013;**6**(9):687-698. DOI: 10.1002/jbio.201200105.

[24] Acar Ö., Özkurt E., Demir G., Saraç H., Alkan C., Esen T., Somel M., Lack N.A. Determining the origin of synchronous multifocal bladder cancer by exome sequencing. BMC Cancer. 2015;**15**(1):871. DOI: 10.1186/s12885-015-1859-8.

[25] Charfi S., Khabir A., Mnif H., Ellouze S., Mhiri M.N., Boudawara-Sellami T. Immunohistochemical expression of HER2 in urothelial bladder carcinoma and its correlation with p53 and p63 expression. J Microscopy Ultrastruct. 2013;**1**(1–2):17-21. DOI: 10.1016/j.jmau.2013.06.001.

[26] Goebell P.J., Groshen S.G., Schmitz-Drager B.J. p53 immunohistochemistry in bladder cancer—a new approach to an old question. Urol Oncol. 2010;**28**(4):377-388. DOI: 10.1016/j.urolonc.2010.03.021.

[27] Shariat S.F., Bolenz C., Godoy G., Fradet Y., Ashfaq R., Karakiewicz P.I., Isbarn H., Jeldres C., Rigaud J., Sagalowsky A.I., Lotan Y. Predictive value of combined immunohistochemical markers in patients with pT1 urothelial carcinoma at radical cystectomy. J Urol. 2009;**182**(1):78-84. DOI: 10.1016/j.juro.2009.02.125.

[28] Yalçin Ö., Sağlican Y., Özdemir S., Özkan N., Mangir N., Eren F. The Relationship of p16, Ki-67, Bcl-2, P53 and CK20 immune expressions with recurrence in superficial bladder tumors. World J Pathol. 2015;**4**:44-51.

[29] Nadkami S.K., Pierce M.C., Park B.H., de Boer J.F., Whittaker P., Bouma B.E., Bressner J.E., Halpern E., Houser S.L., Tearney G.J. Measurement of collagen and smooth muscle cell content in atherosclerotic plaques using polarization-sensitive optical coherence tomography. J Am Coll Cardiol. 2007;**49**(13):1474-1481. DOI: 10.1016/j.jacc.2006.11.040.

[30] Giattina S.D., Courtney B.K., Herz P.R., Harman M., Shortkroff S., Stamper D.L., Liu B., Fujimoto J.G., Brezinski M.E. Assessment of coronary plaque collagen with polarization sensitive optical coherence tomography (PS-OCT). Int J Cardiol. 2006;**107**(3):400-409. DOI: 10.1016/j.ijcard.2005.11.036.

[31] Gubarkova E.V., Kirillin M.Y., Sergeeva E.A., Kiseleva E.B., Snopova L.B., Prodanets N.N., Sharabrin E.G., Shakhov E.B., Nemirova S.V., Gladkova N.D. Cross-polarization optical coherence tomography in evaluation of atherosclerotic plaque structure. Sovrem Tehnol Med. 2013;**5**(4):45-54. DOI: 10.17691/stm2015.7.4.05.

[32] Provenzano P.P., Eliceiri K.W., Campbell J.M., Inman D.R., White J.G., Keely P.J. Collagen reorganization at the tumor-stromal interface facilitates local invasion. BMC Med. 2006;**4**:38. DOI: 10.1186/1741-7015-4-38.

[33] Chrouser K., Leibovich B., Bergstralh E., Zincke H., Blute M. Bladder cancer risk following primary and adjuvant external beam radiation for prostate cancer. J Urol. 2008;**159**(5 Suppl):S7-S11. DOI: 10.1016/j.juro.2008.03.131.

[34] Jacobs B.L., Lee C.T., Montie J.E. Bladder cancer in 2010: how far have we come?. CA Cancer J Clin. 2010;**60**(4):244-272. DOI: 10.3322/caac.20077.

[35] Suriano F, Altobelli E, Sergi F, Buscarini M. Bladder cancer after radiotherapy for prostate cancer. Rev Urol. 2013;**15**(3):108-112.

[36] Dorr W. Radiation effect in normal tissue—principles of damage and protection. Nuklearmedizin. 2010;**49**(1):S53-S58.

[37] Hendry J.H., Jeremic B., Zubizarreta E.H. Normal tissue complications after radiation therapy. Rev Panam Salud Publica. 2006;**20**(2–3):151-160. https://dx.doi.org/10.1590/S1020-49892006000800012.

[38] Cancer Therapy Evaluation Program. Common Terminology Criteria for Adverse Events (CTCAE) v4.0 [Internet]. 2010. [Updated: 2016.08.07]. Available from: https://ctep.cancer.gov/protocoldevelopment/electronic_applications/ctc.htm#ctc_40 [Accessed: 2016.08.10].

[39] Thrasivoulou C., Virich G., Krenacs T., Korom I., Becker D.L. Optical delineation of human malignant melanoma using second harmonic imaging of collagen. Biomed Opt Express. 2011;**2**(5):1282-1295. DOI: 10.1364/BOE.2.001282.

Chapter 4

Bladder Cancer Markers and Recent Innovations

Mariapia Viola-Magni, Samuela Cataldi and
Daniela Marocco

Additional information is available at the end of the chapter

http://dx.doi.org/10.5772/67309

Abstract

Bladder cancer (urothelial carcinoma) is the most common tumor of the urinary tract. It occurs more frequently among men about 65 years old on average. Two forms of the tumor are known: a non–muscle-invasive one and a muscle-invasive one. The latter turns out to be very aggressive with a survival of 5 years average. The non–muscle-invasive form frequently recurs (60–70%) and in 15% of cases, it progresses into the invasive form. The diagnosis is made mainly by cystoscopy and urine cytology. A high number of researches were dedicated in order to find a simple test using voided urine to frequently monitor possible tumor recurrence. During the last 10 years, many tests were proposed concerning either special proteins of which the most common are the bladder tumor antigen (BTA) and the nuclear matrix protein 22 (NMP22) or the presence of genetic mutations [most frequently, fibroblasts growth factor receptor 3 (FGFR3) and TP53], alteration of DNA methylation, chromatin structure and, more recently, the presence of specific micro-RNA. Recently the analysis of lipids present in voided urine showed a difference in fatty acids between healthy individuals and those affected by non-invasive forms. These markers appear to have a high specificity and sensitivity: a deepening of these results could lead to the development of a test that avoids invasive treatment and the cost of cystoscopy.

Keywords: bladder cancer, bladder cancer screening, urinary markers, DNA mutations, lipid metabolism

1. Introduction

1.1. Epidemiology

Urothelial carcinoma of the bladder (BC) is one of the most common urogenital cancers, and according with the American Cancer Society in 2016, it accounts for about 5% of all new cancers in the USA [1]. Chances for men to suffer from BC are three to four times higher than for women. This trend does not seem to be simply due to differences in lifestyle between the sexes (smoke, occupation). Perhaps, women are more protected from this disease than men because estrogen does not stimulate or (maybe) encourage the inhibition of oncogenesis [2]. This fact is supported by both *in vivo* experiments and data concerning mortality incidence [3]. Usually the first diagnosis is performed between 65 and 70 years, but it may occur earlier [2].

1.2. Etiology

Tobacco smoking is the major risk factor for bladder cancer; in fact, smokers develop bladder cancer four times more than non-smokers [4]. Long time smokers have a higher risk of getting sick, and this trend remains even in former smokers up to 20 years [2, 4]. The process that leads to carcinogenesis has not yet been described in detail nor has there been a clear definition as to which of the 60 carcinogens found in tobacco smoke are directly involved with cancer development [5]. However, some free radicals seem to have clear links with tumor development [5]. A linear relationship was found between smoking status and 4-ABPDNA adduct formation and an increase in alterations in p53 tumor suppressor gene (TSG) expression [6]. Metabolism of arylamines are also involved in bladder carcinogenesis. In fact, N-hydroxy metabolites are filtered into the bladder lumen and hit the epithelial tissue, thereby triggering a process of tumorigenesis. The processes of detoxification, catalyzed by *N*-acetyltransferase, are under genetic control. The risk of developing bladder cancer is stronger in individuals with *N*-acetyltransferase-2 slow acetylators. There is a strict relationship between environmental exposure and genetic risk factor [7, 8]. Therefore, the link between smoking and suffering from bladder cancer seems to be weaker than the one between smoking and developing respiratory tract tumors. In fact, there are populations with high smoking rates but low bladder cancer rates [2]. Certain occupational groups are at increased risk of developing bladder cancer because of their chronic exposure to chemical agents. Also, in this case, the probability of developing a bladder tumor depends on an individual susceptibility to this disease [9]. However, some workers mainly employed in textile and tire industries are at increased risk. Several substances, such as naphthylamine, 4-aminobiphenyl (ABP), and benzidine, were unambiguously associated with bladder cancer and are now banned. Other substances such as ortho-toluidine, polychlorinated biphenyls, formaldehyde, asbestos, and solvents such as benzene, dioxane, and methylene chloride are considered strong candidates for bladder carcinogens. Other risk factors for the development of a bladder cancer are chronic infection or irritation of the bladder, which causes an involuntary contraction of the bladder muscles that results in an urgent, uncontrollable need to urinate. A higher possibility of developing genetic mutations is also favored by an increased cell proliferation due to infections and inflammatory processes that favor the formation of nitrite and nitrosamines [2]. The intake of analgesics that contain phenacetin or cyclophosphamide are also correlated with an increased risk of developing urothelial carcinoma. Travis et al. found that the risk of developing bladder cancer following therapy with cyclophosphamide increased by 4.5-fold and was dependent upon a cumulative dose [10]. A study concerning the risk of bladder cancer in women found that radiotherapy in the pelvic area for treatment of ovarian cancer is a potential risk factor [11].

http://dx.doi.org/10.5772/67309

Infection (in the Middle East) with parasites such as *Bilharzia* and *Schistosoma haematobium* is also a known risk factor for bladder cancer [12, 13]. Rare cases of hereditary bladder cancer were found to be related to a mutation in the retinoblastoma tumor suppressor gene [2, 14].

1.3. Pathology

The most common bladder tumors in Western countries are urothelial transitional cell carcinoma (that counts over 90% of total cases), but there are other less common forms of tumor: squamous cell carcinoma, adenocarcinoma and neuroendocrine tumors [4]. Schistosomiasis (*Schistosoma haematobium*), which is endemic in Africa and in the Middle East, causes chronic granulomatous cystitis. This condition favors the development of squamous metaplasia of the transitional epithelium, which can cause squamous cell carcinoma [15]. Adenocarcinoma begins in glandular cells that are found in the lining of the bladder and is a very rare type of bladder cancer [4, 16].

1.4. Staging

Cancer that is in the lining of the bladder is known as non–muscle-invasive bladder cancer (NMIBC), and about 75% of patients show this degree of severity at first diagnosis [4]. These comprise papillary tumors designated Ta (urothelial) and T1 (extending into the lamina propria) or carcinoma *in situ* (CIS), a flat erythematous lesion with a propensity to progress to muscle-invasive disease (MIBC). This is a very aggressive cancer with a life expectancy of around 5 years. In fact, during stages T2–T4, the cancer spreads to the muscle layer of the bladder, invades the muscle wall of the bladder, and then disseminates to nearby organs and lymph nodes [4, 16].

Since 2002, a universal staging system can be used, namely, the TNM classification (tumor, lymph nodes, and metastasis). It is very important to be able to define a classification system that is easy to use and reproducible, because it can be crucial to adopt the most appropriate therapy and to predict prognosis [2].

1.5. Signs and symptoms

In most cases, lower urinary tract symptoms and hematuria are the most common early symptoms (85% of patients). Other symptoms include changes in bladder habits, increase in urinary frequency, bladder irritability, and dysuria. Symptoms of advanced bladder cancer are weight loss, abdominal pain, and renal impairment secondary to ureteric obstruction [2].

1.6. Bladder cancer diagnosis and surveillance

Cystoscopy is a diagnostic procedure to examine directly the bladder and is considered the current gold standard for diagnosis and surveillance [4]. This type of examination allows for a possible biopsy that can provide important information about tumors regarding the different developmental stages [17]. It has the disadvantage of expense and is rather invasive. Nevertheless, bladder cancer has a very high cost per patient because NMIBCs have a low progression rate, but are characterized by a high recurrence rate (50–70% within 5 years). For this reason, patients need frequent and expensive surveillance protocols [18, 19]. Despite a correct treatment, some patients may develop muscle-invasive disease that has a high malignant potential and is associated with considerable progression and cancer death rates.

A chemical dipstick for hematuria offers another diagnostic test. Unfortunately, hematuria from bladder cancer may be intermittent, and it occurs also in people who do not have bladder cancer. Furthermore, the detection of the disease may be uncertain and may require repetitive screening [2]. Intravenous urography (IVU) is a diagnostic test in patients with hematuria. It is very specific for upper tract surveillance and diagnosis while the early detection of small urothelial tumors may be particularly difficult to visualize.

Computed tomography (CT) scanning is useful to identify lesions within the ureter, renal pelvis, and renal parenchyma, but is not specific.

Urine-based cytology is more useful for patients who have a history of urinary tract cancer. This test may be ordered to screen patients who are at high risk for bladder cancer and as an adjunct in long-term surveillance protocols [2, 17].

1.7. Urine cytology

Urine cytology is the most commonly used diagnostic technique in clinical practice. Recently, more research on other urine-based markers has been done [20].

Urinary cytopathology is a test used to detect bladder cancer and inflammatory diseases of the urinary tract. It is based on the interpretation of morphological changes in disaggregated cells. Even in the presence of a negative cystoscopic examination, morphological changes such as increased size, increased nuclear-to-cytoplasmic ratio, nuclear pleomorphism, coarse and irregular chromatin ,and frequent mitotic figures are features associated with a higher risk for bladder cancer [18, 21]. This kind of analysis requires a professionally trained and experienced cytopathologist. Incorrect sample collection and processing can adversely affect the accuracy of the results [2]. The possibility of obtaining false positive is very high with intravesical therapy, radiation treatment, and infection, which are able to alter the results [18].

This method is not suitable for screening patients because it is not very sensitive in the cases of low-grade tumors. In fact, it is not easy to identify tumor cells in urine specimens of patients with noninvasive low-grade carcinoma. These cells have particular characteristics that are not always similar to the malignant tumor cells. The early stage, dysplasia, is characterized by the formation of flat, fibrovascular stalks that cannot be identified as neoplastic formations in histological sections.

Urinary cytology is mainly indicated for the detection of high-grade and high-stage disease that shows more recognizable features (nuclear pleomorphism, coarsely clumped chromatin, and large nucleoli) [2]. In fact, urinary cytological analysis can detect carcinoma *in situ* (CIS) with a sensitivity of 80–90% and a specificity of 98–100% because it consists of cells that are significantly abnormal. Urinary cytology can be used in long-term surveillance programs, but it is an expensive technique [18].

http://dx.doi.org/10.5772/67309

1.8. Biomarkers in bladder cancer

The correct treatment of patients with bladder cancer requires an early and accurate diagnosis, which is followed by long-term surveillance. Currently, the most effective tests that could diagnose and monitor the progression of the disease are cystoscopic examination, cytology, and histology. These techniques have promoted a dramatic decrease in the mortality associated with the disease, but they are inadequate for several reasons. They do not allow us to understand the molecular mechanisms underlying the tumor in question; the possibility of human error is quite high; they are expensive and, in the case of cystoscopy, invasive [17].

In recent years, due to improved molecular biology techniques, new classes of diagnostic and prognostic biomarkers have been identified. They have taken into account not only individual proteins but also the interactions between molecules in pathways known to be tumorigenic [22].

Tumorigenesis occurs often with a clear involvement of distinct pathways that can lead to the development of NMIBC or of MIBC. This feature can be used to find out new markers which are able to highlight the pathway involved and, hence, the type of tumor. The study of gene expression in bladder cancer is another type of investigation that is developing [17]. Identifying the ideal marker is not a simple task. Indeed, it needs to feature many requirements together: high sensitivity and specificity, the ability to predict the degree of tumor malignancy, lack of susceptibility to human errors, user-friendliness, noninvasiveness, and price convenience. It should not be influenced by the presence concurrently of other diseases and by the presence of hematuria or irritative symptoms that often occur in patients with bladder cancer [20]. An ideal biomarker should be also able to identify, in a clear way, the disease before its clinical manifestation and, at the same time, to provide accurate prognostic information [17, 23]. By developing non-invasive molecular assays which are able to analyze body fluids, it would be easier to perform a large-scale screening of individuals most at risk [20, 22]. It would be important to be able to develop a test that can express a very strict diagnosis, which allows patient treatment in a personalized way. This ideal marker could relieve the inconvenience inherent in the use of invasive procedures to strictly necessary cases. In the last few years, the aging of the population has caused a dramatic rise in diseases related to age. The incidence of bladder cancer has increased by 36%. This is another reason why it would be useful to have an effective screening method, as is the case for the screening of prostate and colon cancer [20].

The following discussion illustrates the current diagnostic assays for bladder cancer and discusses some of the emerging biomarkers. Some of these studies are at a preliminary stage, but they appear to deserve further investigation and a mention in this text.

2. Current diagnostic assays

2.1. Urine-based assay

2.1.1. Bladder tumor antigen (BTA) assay

The original bladder tumor antigen (BTA) test is an agglutination assay that measures the level of a membrane protein that is released into the urine when the cancer invades the bladder wall.

The BTA test can be used for the detection of low-grade disease and shows a higher sensitivity than cytology. Unfortunately, it cannot be used in patients affected by other disorders such as urinary infections, stones, or benign prostatic hypertrophy (BPH). In such cases, the presence of concomitant diseases can lead to false-positive results [20]. To overcome this lack of precision, two other BTA tests were developed: BTA STAT and BTA TRAK. Both are immunoassays that can detect factor H–related protein (cFH), which is released into the urine by tumor cells [2, 18, 20].

BTA STAT is a qualitative dipstick test [24]. This assay has several advantages: it is fast, is inexpensive, and works with only a few drops of urine. The sensitivity is higher than either the original version of the test or cytology. The results are more accurate in cases of high-grade bladder cancers. Unfortunately, this test has the same problems as the original version. False-positive results are quite common with rates of 2–5%. This assay cannot be used in patients with dysuria, incontinence, and hematuria [20]. Also in the case of bacillus Calmette-Guérrin (BCG) instillation in patients has led to a sharp drop in its accuracy, even if the treatment was made 2 years before. For this reason, BTA STAT cannot be used for the monitoring of the disease in patients who have undergone immunotherapy [20, 22]. The reasons for its low specificity yet its high sensitivity are still not clear. The use of BTA STAT was approved by the U.S. Food and Drug Administration (FDA). However, a constant monitoring of patients is recommended also through cystoscopy. Hence, this technique is not definitive for diagnosis, but it is only indicative [20, 24].

BTA TRAK is a quantitative assay: an ELISA test that detects levels of cFH [20, 22]. The cFH protein can be detected also in case of bladder bleeding [22]. Furthermore, other studies argue that cFH is definitely produced and secreted by the Kupffer cells, hepatocytes, vascular endothelial cells, and platelets, but it has not been proven that bladder cancer cells secrete cFH [22, 25]. The BTA TRAK test shows a higher sensitivity than does either the BTA STAT test or cytology also for the detection of low-grade tumors. However, this test presents problems of low specificity for the same reasons as the BTA test. For this reason, also this test cannot replace urine cytology or cystoscopy. An increase of the test values is often related to the possibility of the development of a recurrence. BTA TRAK may be useful for quantifying the correct time interval between the cystoscopic analyses individually in a patient with a recurrence, but this assumption needs further work [20].

2.1.2. Nuclear matrix protein 22 (NMP22)

Nuclear matrix proteins (NMPs) have a structural role in cellular nuclei and are involved in DNA replication, transcription, RNA processing, and gene expression. In particular, NMP22 is a specific protein of the nuclear matrix that is involved in the correct distribution of the genetic material to daughter cells during mitosis [20]. Two different texts to detect this protein have been developed: NMP22 test, which is a quantitative immunoassay and NMP22 BladderChek, which is a qualitative point-of-care test. Apoptosis causes the release of this protein into the urine that can be detected using monoclonal antibodies. Urine of patients with bladder cancer contains a greater amount of this protein compared to healthy controls [2, 18, 20]. Thus, this test provides a measure of cell turnover. The sensitivity is about 51–85% and increases with the support of cytology [18]. Also other bladder diseases affect the reliability of this test negatively and the rate of false positive is quite high [20, 24]. NMP22 is not suitable to be used for screening exams; however, some studies have found positive correlations between NMP22 levels and the aggressiveness of the cancer. This correlation can be exploited to make assessments on patient prognosis [20, 26, 27]. The evaluation of NMP22 levels may also have predictive value for the risk of recurrence. In fact, Soloway et al. found that patients who exceed a threshold value of NMP22 level (20 U/ml) have a greater probability to develop a recurrence [28].

2.1.3. BLCA-1 and BLCA-4

BladderCancer-1/BladderCancer-4 (BLCA-1 and BLCA-4) are members of six bladder-specific nuclear matrix proteins (NMPs) discovered in 1996 by Getzenberg et al. [29]. These proteins are involved in important cellular functions such as DNA replication and RNA synthesis and in nuclear morphology [30]. Many NMPs are identified as specific markers for several cancers [31]. BLCA-1 and BLCA-4 are considered specific urinary markers of bladder cancer. In particular, they are associated with tumor cell proliferation, survival, and angiogenesis [29–31]. The expression of these factors is important to detect bladder cancer at an early stage, since they are expressed early in carcinogenesis [18]. BLCA-1 was originally identified from bladder tumor tissue, while BLCA-4 is expressed in both tumor and adjacent benign areas of the bladder, but not in bladders without malignancy [29, 30]. Probably they play different roles in the regulation of the gene expression in bladder cancer [32]. Although BCL-1 has high sensitivity and specificity while its role is not yet clear in the development of bladder cancer. BCL-4 has sensitivity and specificity higher than other urinary tumor markers. The detection BCL-4 expression is not affected by the presence benign bladder disorders but may increase in patients with spinal cord injuries. Both BCL-1 and BLCA-4 assays still need further refinement and validation if they are to be included into clinical practice [30].

2.1.4. Urinary Bladder Cancer test (UBC)

Cytokeratins (CKs) are intracellular proteins in the intracytoplasmic cytoskeleton of epithelial cells. They are overexpressed in bladder cancer and are released into the urine as soluble fragments after proteolytic degradation following cell death [18, 33]. Because of such features, various assays measuring the concentration of soluble cytokeratins, such as TPS for cytokeratin 18 and TPA for cytokeratin 8, 18, and 19, have been used to detect bladder tumors [34]. Immunological assays UBC-Rapid and UBC-ELISA tests are used to detect the concentration of a combination of cytokeratin 8 and 18 fragments [18]. The **UBC-Rapid test** is a qualitative point-of-care assay that shows a high variability of sensitivities and specificities that probably is due to the histological and clinical characteristics of bladder cancer [18, 33]. This assay requires no special knowledge as the case of BTA STAT and is more sensitive and specific. However, it has a low sensitivity in the detection of bladder cancer recurrence and cannot replace, but only lower, the number of cystoscopies heeded during the patient's follow-up [35–37]. **UBC-ELISA** is a quantitative assay. It is limited by a strong possibility of human error and it is characterized by a high variability of sensitivity and specificity, a high false-positive rates and the inability to detect low-grade tumors. Further studies are needed to assess their potential diagnostic role and to increase the utility of these tests for bladder tumor surveillance [18].

2.1.5. CYFRA 21-1

Cytokeratin Fragments (CYFRA 21-1) is also an ELISA-based assay that detects the concentration of soluble fragments of cytokeratin using two mouse monoclonal antibodies. Various studies on the sensitivity and specificity of the assay have reported different results. Possible reasons include the different tumor grade of the patient populations and the differences in the method of urine collection and storage [34]. The centrifugation step is very important to remove cells and cell debris that contains a large amount of CYFRA 21-1, though the accuracy of the assay is not improved yet. In fact, after centrifugation an equivalent decrease in the number of true positive and false positive can be observed [38]. CYFRA 21-1 is found at high concentrations in the urine of patients with benign diseases of the bladder. Also intravesical immunotherapy with BCG increased concentrations of urinary CYFRA 21-1, even after years of treatment, when there was no evidence of a bladder tumor. This assay has a high sensitivity for the detection of high-grade and CIS tumors, but it cannot be used for early detection. This assay shows greater accuracy for the detection of primary tumors than for the recurrence. Currently, it cannot be used as a substitute for cystoscopy and has achieved only an arguable and marginal role in daily clinical practice [34].

2.1.6. Survivin

Survivin is a member of the inhibitors of apoptosis proteins (IAP) gene family that is involved in apoptosis inhibition [39]. Survivin is expressed during embryonic and fetal development but not in normal adult tissues. It is also abundantly expressed in transformed cells and in many tumors. Survivin promotes an abnormal elongation of cell life that leads to an accumulation of genetic mutations and can promote resistance to immune-surveillance. Researchers are interested in exploiting the information on survivin for diagnostic and clinical purposes. For this reason, they are studying its role as a promoter of carcinogenesis but also the pathways in which it is involved. The detection of survivin in the urine is obtained by a BioDot microfiltration detection system. Dots of the urine samples are blotted on nitrocellulose membranes and survivin can be detected using various anti-survivin antibodies and standard dot blot detection reagents [40]. Survivin has a high sensitivity for detecting low-stage and low-grade bladder tumors often underdiagnosed by other diagnostic tests. High level of the urine's survivin is associated with increased risk of bladder cancer, of tumors of higher grade, and of bladder cancer recurrence. This assay is more accurate than cytology tests using urine. Moreover, it is also more accurate than NMP22 tests and avoids false-positive results.

Survivin is present in the urine of 78% of patients with localized disease. Its level could be skewed in patients with either T1 or higher tumor stage than in patients with Ta disease or CIS. Its use in the diagnosis would require further evaluation and a deepening study of the signaling pathways in the bladder cancer [41].

http://dx.doi.org/10.5772/67309

2.2. Cell-based assay

2.2.1. ImmunoCyt/uCyt+ assay

Fradet and Lockhard developed the immunofluorescence-based test ImmunoCyt/uCyt+ in 1997. These are two markers that are expressed in malignant exfoliated urothelial cells and few normal umbrella cells and are not found in the other normal cells [17, 18, 42]. This assay uses a cocktail of three antibodies: the first antibody (19A211) is directed against a glycosylated carcinoembryonic antigen and is labeled red; the other two antibodies, M344 and LDQ10, labeled with fluorescein, are directed against mucins [18, 42]. The mucins are glycoproteins that are normally found on the surface of epithelial cells. In normal cells, these glycoproteins are found in heavily glycosylated form while in malignant cells these glycoproteins are less glycosylated. This test uses LDQ10 and M344 antibodies that can recognize some portions of the protein backbone [42]. The recognition of the results is given a lot to the cythopathologist's skill. In fact, to have a negative response, cytology slide should contain at least 500 cells that are negative for fluorescence while the presence of one fluorescent cell is considered to be positive. This assay is not very influenced by factors such hematuria or inflammatory conditions because it is a cellular assay. ImmunoCyt/uCyt+ has a superior sensitivity to detect early pathological stage than cytology. It can also improve the detection of CIS and increase the sensitivity of the urinary cytology [18]. However, to be valid, this assay must always be accompanied by cytological analysis, and it is only suitable for the surveillance of patients with a history of bladder cancer [18, 42].

A combination of multiple immunological tests is considered useful for diagnosis and prognosis. Recently a combination of p40, GATA3, and uroplakin II (transmembrane protein) antibody has been proposed [43].

2.2.2. UroVysion fluorescence in situ hybridization (FISH)

UroVysion is also a fluorescence-based assay. It was developed in 2000 and is FDA approved as a urine marker for the diagnosis and the surveillance of bladder cancer [24]. Exfoliated urothelial cells are analysed exploiting the technique of fluorescence *in situ* hybridization (FISH) to detect the aneuploidy of chromosomes 3, 7, and 17 and loss of the 9p21 locus [17, 18]. As the case of ImmunoCyt/uCyt+ assay, this assay is quite complex and requires the interpretation of a skilled cytopathologist. In fact, the result is considered to be positive if either at least five cells are found with two extra chromosomes, or ten cells with an extra chromosome, or a homozygous deletion of 9p21 in >20% of the epithelial cells [24]. UroVysion has a higher sensitivity in diagnosis or recurrence of bladder cancer than other types of analysis. A positive result of UroVysion test, in patients who have been previously treated with BCG, can warn doctors about treatment failure. Unfortunately, this assay has the disadvantages of providing many false-positive results and is found to be more sensitive in cases of high-grade tumor than in case of low-grade disease. Thus, it is recommended to use UroVysion after ImmunoCyt/uCyt+ test or cytological analysis as a confirmatory test [18, 44].

2.2.3. DD23

DD23 is an IgG murine monoclonal antibody (MAb) derived from the immunization of a BALB/c mouse that recognizes a 185-kDa tumor-associated antigen. This antigen is not detected in normal urothelium while it is expressed in human bladder cancer cells, both *in vitro* and *in vivo* [45]. However, a study observed that in patients with bladder cancer, DD23 antigen is expressed in cancerous as well as in noncancerous cells. One theory holds that normal urothelial cells in response to external signals from the malignant cells express DD23 [45, 46]. This immune-cytochemical assay is performed using an avidin-biotin alkaline phosphatase, with a single urothelial cell exhibiting intense immunostaining sufficient to make a positive call. However, there are various methods of DD23 detection [47]. For example, Bonner et al. used a highly sensitive automated quantitative fluorescence image analysis system, whereas Gilbert et al. used a commercial clinical reference laboratory-adapted qualitative immunocytochemistry assay with light-based microscopy [45, 46]. The cytological analysis of urine sediment carried out using murine IgG1 monoclonal antibody (MAb) together with Papanicolaou (Pap) staining is difficult both from practical use and from an interpretative point of view. Even this technique has a higher sensitivity for the detection of high-grade tumors than low-grade ones [47–52]. DD23 antigen expression must be supported by cytological analysis. It can enhance the sensitivity of the cytopathology diagnosis of 21%, especially in low-grade cancers and can increase the detection of unclassified TCC cases [45, 53, 54]. This assay is not very suitable for the detection of recurrence in patients who have previously received an intravesical therapy. DD23 can be a support of cystoscopic examination to increase the sensitivity to monitor and diagnosis recurrent bladder cancer. The use of this biomarker needs further clinical studies [45].

These assays are summarized in **Table 1** with their characteristics.

	Sensitivity	Specificity	Limitations
Urine-based assay			
BTA STAT	53–83%	67–72%	High false-positive rates.
BTA TRAK	66–72%	51–75%	High false-positive rate.
Nuclear matrix protein 22 (NMP22)	51–85%	77–96%	False positive in case of hematuria or inflammatory bladder conditions.
BLCA-1	80%	87%	It needs futher validation.
BLCA-4	89–96%	90–100%	It needs futher validation.
UBC-Rapid test	36–78%	63–97%	High variability of sensitivities and specificities. Hight false-positive rate. Low sensitivity in the detection of low-grade bladder tumors.
UBC-ELISA	40–70%	63–75%	Hight false-positive rate. Low sensitivity in the detection of low-grade bladder tumors.
CYFRA 21-1	61–85%	75–91%	False positive in case of inflammatory bladder conditions.
Survivin	64–83%	88–93%	It needs futher validation.

http://dx.doi.org/10.5772/67309

	Sensitivity	Specificity	Limitations
Cell-based assay			
ImmunoCyt/uCyt+ assay	68%	72%	The test results depend on specimen stability and handling.
UroVysion fluorescence *in situ* hybridization (FISH)	69–75%	82–85%	Low sensitivity in the detection of low-grade bladder tumors. Lack of consensus regarding criteria used to evaluate abnormal cells.
DD23 (*)	70.3%	59.8%	It can be used as an adjunct to cytopathologic evaluation.

All the data derived from Ref. [17], except (*) from Ref. [23].

Table 1. Sensitivity and specificity of urine-based and cell-based assays.

3. Nucleic acids alterations

Circulating DNA has been demonstrated in all body fluids, including urine, and it is the demonstration of many tumor-related alterations, particularly for colon cancer. For this reason, many researches were made on urine and bladder samples in order to analyze free DNA and RNA fragments present. An increase in DNA was found in both the voided urine and plasma of patients with NMIBC with respect to non-affected patients [55]. Aggressive tumors show very high DNA values. Analysis of the DNA may represent a novel diagnostic tool to indicate the presence of residual disease or to discover aggressive forms early in the bladder cancer course. Analysis of the DNA showed 302 mutations of exons, 204 segmental alterations in genomic copy number. and 22 genomic rearrangements for a given sample [56]. Three different groups were identified based on the gene alterations. Group A, classified as focally amplified, is enriched in focal somatic mutations in many genes; group B is characterized by CDKN2A-deficient fibroblast growth factor receptor 3 (FGFR3) mutant defined papillary from the histological aspect; and group C, classified as "tumor protein p53 (TP53) cell-cycle mutant", is enriched with RB1 mutations and amplifications of E2F3and CCNI [56].

It has been suggested that these differences may represent different oncogenic mechanisms. In non-invasive tumors, mutations were found especially in the oncogenes Harvey rat sarcoma (HRAS), fibroblasts growth factor receptor 3 (FGFR3), and phosphatidylinositol-3-kinase (PK3CA).

In invasive tumors, mutations have been found in tumor suppressor genes, especially TP53 and retinoblastoma (RB1) [57]. The presence of the FGFR3 mutation in urine is observed for low-grade tumors and seems to be associated with concomitant or future recurrence [57, 58]. Methylation is also important: five targets were identified, including ventral and anterior homeobox 1 (WAX1) KCNV1, TAL1, PPOX1, and CFTR, which have a sensitivity of 88.68% and a specificity of 87.25%. An increase in methylation is also observed for the tumor suppressor gene RUNX3 gene [59, 60]. In particular, methylation of VAX1 and LMX1A appears to be associated with bladder cancer recurrence. Promoter hypermethylation of some genes combined with FGFR3 mutations may represent a sensitive diagnostic assay [61]. Methylation of the tumor suppressor gene H-cadherin (CDH13) has been reported in many cancers, and an increase is observed especially in Asian patients affected by bladder cancer [62]. The CDH13 gene, located on 16q24, encodes a protein that belongs to the cadherin family [63]. CDH13, a tumor suppressor gene (TSG), is also called H-cadherin or T-cadherin and plays a pivotal role in cell–cell adhesion [64]. The expression of this gene favors the adhesion between the cells, thus inhibiting metastatic diffusion.

3.1. Microsatellite analysis

Microsatellites (or short tandem repeats) are repeated noncoding DNA sequences consisting of very short repeat units (mostly 2–4 bp each) arranged in a tandem repeat. They can be used as molecular markers of loci and play an essential role in the structure of chromosomes. Two types of microsatellite alteration are involved in many cancers: loss of heterozygosity due to a deletion and genomic instability due to an alteration of microsatellite repeat length [40, 65].

Several studies have been published on the correlation between microsatellite alterations in bladder transitional cell carcinoma (TCC). In particular, they have observed 17 microsatellite loci. The loci on chromosomes 9 and 18 have proven to be the most informative [66–69]. Saidi et al. compared two microsatellite loci (GSN and/or D18S51) of patients with histopathologically confirmed bladder TCC, with normal bladder mucosa and with non-malignant diseases. They found alterations in 46 out of 70 patients with TCC, but none in the tissue samples from the control group [70]. This analysis showed a sensitivity of 65.71%, and specificity of 100% but, according to the literature data, frequency of microsatellite alterations in urinary bladder TCC varies a great deal [67, 70, 71]. Unfortunately, microsatellite analysis is time-consuming, expensive, and requires highly trained personnel. Furthermore, Saidi et al. have not found a close correlation between the pathological stages as recurrence, metastasis, and death, in patients with TCC, followed by at least 2 years [70]. The study of the possible use of microsatellites as a tumor marker is complicated also by other point of view: the correct selection of microsatellite loci, their polymorphic nature and ethnic differences in patient populations are features that affect the results between studies [70, 72].

4. Chromatin alterations

Mutations in chromatin could lead to alterations in genes involved in human carcinomas [73]. In high-grade bladder cancer over 2300 alterations were found as well as in genes involving chromatin modifiers [74]. This implies that epigenetic modulators could have a therapeutic role in urothelial cancers [73]. Varticovski et al. performed comparative bio-informatic analysis on mutations in several previously identified genes associated with bladder cancer. They found mutations in TP53, RAS, and TERT genes and mutations/deletions in several chromatin modifiers KDM6A and MLL2/3. They found also mutations in novel sites distant from promoters showing a reprogramming of regulatory networks. Many of these mutations occur in characteristic sites unique for each stage of the tumor progression. This feature has potential clinical application providing valuable new information on bladder cancer biology and tumor progression [74]. The coiling of DNA around nucleosome particles is the basis of genome organization with histone modifications being associated with both active and repressed regions of chromatin. Acetylation or phosphorylation may change the chromatin structure by altering the net positive charge of the histone proteins so changing the accessibility of the underlying information sequences. Modifications of histones are reported for many tumors and are correlated to tumor stage and prognosis, but with contradicting results [75]. Histone acetylation is catalyzed by a specific enzyme family, histone acetyltransferases (HATs), and correlates with nucleosome remodelling and transcriptional activation, whereas deacetylation of histone tails is catalyzed by histone deacetylases (HDACs) induces transcriptional repression through chromatin condensation [76]. Altered expression of different HDACs has been reported inr various human cancers [77–83]. Bladder tumor chemotherapies, which act as inhibitor of acetyltransferase, have shown that the decrease in tumor cellular growth *in vitro* is due to the acetylation of histone lysine with a consequent imbalance between histone acetylation and de-acetylation.

4.1. Telomerase

The telomere is the terminal region of eukaryotic chromosome and is composed of highly repetitive DNA sequences (e.g., TTAGGG in humans). It was thought to be a non-coding region while recent discoveries have speculated that it is involved in the regulation of telomerase. Telomerase is a ribonucleoprotein organized to form a complex that includes: an RNA component, human telomerase RNA (hTR), and telomerase reverse transcriptase (hTERT) that is a catalytic protein. In normal cells, DNA polymerase is not able to replicate the chromosome until its termination. In fact, after each DNA replication, there is a progressive shortening of chromosomes with a consequent loss of genetic information, which causes chromosomal instability and cellular senescence. Telomerase maintains telomere length in several cancer cells types [40]. It keeps intact chromosomes adding telomeres at the ends chromosomes, lengthening again the shortened telomeres. In normal cells it is active only during embryonic development while in most normal adult tissues its expression is repressed [84]. The expression of telomerase in tumor cells immortalize them [85]. This mechanism can be considered a crucial step in tumorigenesis [84].

The telomeric repeat amplification protocol (TRAP) assay is used to measure telomerase activity. Telomerase reaction products are detectable by several commercial kits that provide optimized sets of primers and reagents for telomerase detection. Another method allows measurement of hTERT mRNA levels by RT-PCR. The sensitivity of these assays is variable: it depends on sample manipulation but also on the presence of inflammatory conditions that can contaminate benign cells with telomerase activity [86–96]. The specificity of both the TRAP assay and hTERT RT-PCR is also variable. Telomerase assays are not suitable for use in clinical settings. To overcome these problems, it requires more clinical trials [40].

5. RNA messenger

The detection of (*hTERT*), mRNA of human telomerase reverse transcriptase, using RT-PCR was considered as a valid tool for a noninvasive tumor diagnosis test. However, in urine we can found a significant amounts of cell-free RNA and for this reason RNA tumor markers (e.g., *hTERT, UPK1A, HTATIP2*), cannot be used unconditionally for RT-qPCR–based analysis of whole urine [97]. Another system that has been intensively studied for its role in tumorigenesis is *uPA*: *ETS2*. The *uPA* promoter region contains *ETS2* binding sites, a member of the *ETS* family of transcription factors. *uPA* mRNA content in tissue and urinary protein concentrations of uPA are suitable for bladder cancer diagnostics. In the case of bladder cancer higher *ETS2* RNA concentration it is observed compared with *uPA*. This tumor marker ratio of *ETS2*: *uPA* could be an interesting diagnostic tool [97–101]. Hedegaard et al. prepared a total RNA-sequencing (RNA-seq) libraries for 476 patients with bladder cancer at different stages (Ta, T1, *in situ* [CIS], MIBC). They mapped sequences to the human genome and then explored the heterogeneity in early-stage bladder cancer of 8074 genes [102]. The results were interpreted by statistical analysis and, on the basis of these results; the bladder tumors were sub-grouped into three major classes [102–104]. They found that tumors of high stage and grade were more frequently observed in classes 2 and 3 than in class 1.

Particularly, MIBC and high-risk NMIBC were more frequently observed in the same cluster 2 showing similarities. Differences in gender or smoking status do not influence the results [102]. Class 3 tumors show basal-like characteristics. They are mainly associated with repressed genes and with modifications of histones and/or chromatin. Class 1 tumors are characterized by a good prognosis, while class 2 shows poor prognosis and high expression of late cell-cycle genes, which have previously been associated with aggressiveness in bladder cancer [102, 105, 106]. Class 1 and class 2 tumors display different levels of aggressiveness. This study can be overlapped with other previous studies [105]. This kind of analysis could be a way for optimized surveillance programs and treatment selection [102].

6. Micro RNA

Micro RNA are short non-coding RNAs (18–25 nucleotides) that can change the expression of mRNA. This kind of regulation can take place directly by interaction with mRNA, by translation regulation of the protein product or by mRNA degradation. A single miRNA can regulate multiple genes or more miRNA can be involved in a single target (**Figure 1**) [107].

They can, therefore, regulate the expression of many genes and the analysis of these molecules may be important for understanding many biological processes such as epithelial to mesenchymal transition, which is a relevant mechanism in bladder cancer tumor development. Micro RNAs are present in many body fluids including urine, are resistant to RNase

http://dx.doi.org/10.5772/67309

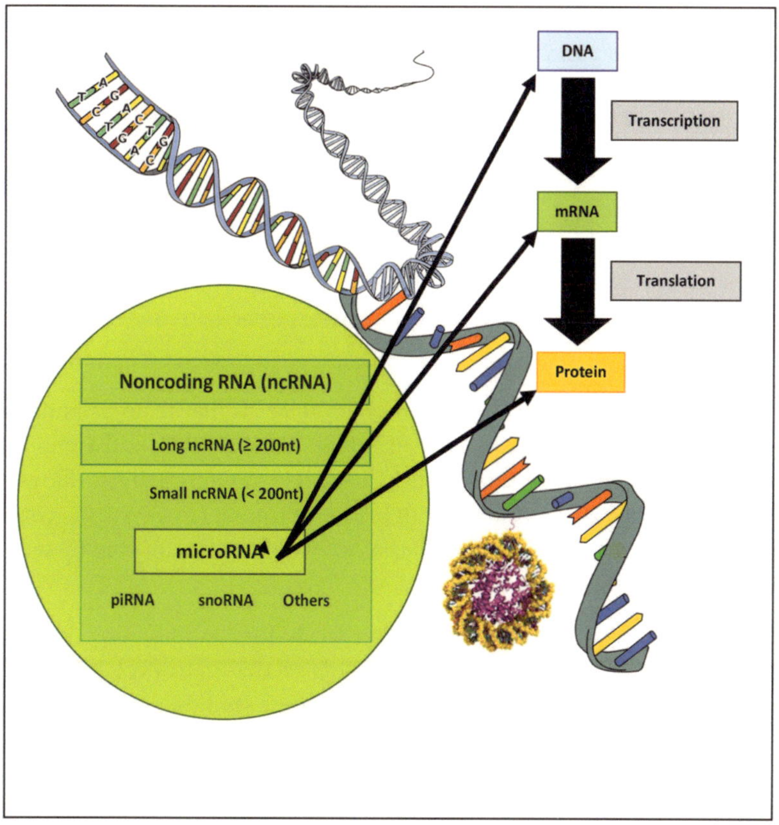

Figure 1. Functions of mi-RNA.

and also can be preserved for long time, so they can be determined using non-invasive methods. Many miRNAs were found in the urine, some of them might be correlated with renal or prostatic diseases, as well as bladder cancer [108].

Recently, a list of miRNAs detected in bladder cancer as well as their target genes has been reported. At the moment, a complete analysis is unavailable, but some results indicate some differences in relation to bladder cancer, particularly in relation to their invasiveness and prognosis.

An increase of miR 21, the cluster miR 183-96-1, miR 210, and miR 205 is observed to influence the epithelial-mesenchymal transition, cell growth and migration. On the other hand, a decrease is observed in many others, like miR 29c, miR 124, miR 409, miRs 23 family, miRs-200 family, miR-214, that favors apoptosis and inhibit cell proliferation. miR-205 discriminates between low-grade papillary urothelial carcinoma and high grade papillary urothelial carcinoma, whereas miR-145 distinguished high-grade papillary urothelial carcinoma from infiltrating carcinoma [109]. The increase of the expression levels of miR-200c and miR-141 in patients with bladder cancer after surgical removal of the tumor appears to return to normal values [110]; miR-126, miR-182, and miR-199a are the most abundant in the urine of bladder cancer patients with respect to the controls [107]. Ratios of miR-12 s6/miR-152 and miR-182/miR-152 are considered as makers capable of distinguishing bladder cancer patients from controls and patients affected by infections. Their sensitivity and specificity are not very high ranging from 55 to 82%. Yamada et al. found that the detection of miR-96 in the urine has a sensitivity of 71.8% and a specificity of 89.2% [111]. Shimizu et al. reported also good specificity and sensitivity by testing a methylation panel of miR9-3, miR124-2, miR124-3, and miR 137 [112]. As regards to a prognostic evaluation, miR2103, miR214, miR152, and miR3187-3p are predicting a recurrence-free survival [113–115].

7. Proteins

Proteomics analysis allows the identification of proteins in the urine of patients. Some of these proteins such as alpha-defensin, apolipoprotein A-1 (APOA1), and alpha-1-antitrypsin are present in increased levels in tumor cells [116]. Metabolomic analysis allowed the identification of some metabolites associated with bladder tumors. However, the correct association of the results with a type of tumor can be difficult to establish due to small molecule renal filtration.

There are several proteins that are worth further study for evaluation as new possible biomarkers. **Fibronectin** is a multifunctional, extracellular matrix glycoprotein. It is produced by a wide variety of cells and is present in many tissues. Some studies have shown that increases in the urine content in case of the bladder cancer [117–119]. **Clusterin** is a heterodimeric disulfide-linked glycoprotein, implicated in a number of biological processes. It is a chaperone protein present in two isoforms (1 and 2) with antagonistic actions exhibiting different cellular locations. Clusterin gene increases its expression in bladder cancer particularly in invasive disease [120]. High clusterin expression is associated with poor prognosis. However, it is expressed in all body fluids and this feature limited its specificity. It would be necessary to detect the individual expression of the two isoform rather than total clusterin levels [121]. Tilki et al. reported **CEACAM1** (Carcinoembryonic antigen-related cell adhesion molecule 1, also known as CD66a) as a novel urinary marker for bladder cancer. Sensitivity was higher for MIBC than NMIBC and thougth patients with diabetes were excluded from the study. Furthermore, CEACAM1 immunostaining disappears in urothelium of NMIBC while appears in adjacent tumor-associated endothelial cells [122]. **Calprotectin** is a protein with antimicrobial properties [123]. It was suggested as a prognostic indicator because it results in upregulation in bladder cancer with 80% sensitivity at 92% specificity [124, 125]. However, it is released also by neutrophils during inflammatory processes and this feature compromises its accuracy [126]. **Stathmin-1** and **CD147** are two urinary proteins studied for their correlation with bladder cancer. In fact, there are reports that overexpression of stathmin-1 and CD147 are associated with aggressive bladder cancer and a poor prognosis [127, 128]. **γ-synuclein** is involved in the pathogenesis of neurodegenerative diseases and is also used as a marker in breast tumors. It shows 87.5% sensitivity and 90.0% specificity. **DJ-1** has been reported to be overexpressed in aggressive high-grade bladder cancer [129]. A pilot study found urinary DJ-1 to be significantly increased only in MIBC [130]. The specificity of **Apolipoprotein A4 for bladder** cancer is not confirmed even if various apolipoproteins increase in the urine of bladder cancer patients [131]. In Kumar et al probably was overestimated the presence **coronin-1A** (a cytoskeletal protein) in urine of patient with bladder cancer [130, 132]. Orenes-Piñero et al. realized an immunohistochemistry analysis, followed a proteomics analysis, that showed Reg-1 (lithostathine-1-alpha) overexpression in bladder tumors [133]. Urinary levels of matrix metallopeptidase 9 (**MMP9**) are elevated in many cases of invasive bladder cancer. However, it shows a modest sensitivity and specificity in case of low-grade disease [134–141]. The majority of the biomarker studies could not be classified as unequivocal. This conclusion may be due to a loss of information (stage/grade/sensitivity/specificity) or due to a non-representative patient population that overstates the sensitivity and specificity [130].

8. Lipids

There have been very few published analyses of lipids as potential biomarkers, although an increase in the serum of lipids and proteins associated with sialic acid were demonstrated to differentiate patients from healthy control groups, showing a sensitivity of around 80% and a specificity of 70% [142]. A rare variant of urothelial carcinoma has been characterized by large epithelial cells with an eccentric nucleus and vacuolated cytoplasm that resemble lipoblasts, which are also positive for cytokeratin 7, 20, CAM 5.2, and other proteins. Only in one publication on bladder tissue has the composition of fatty acids been taken into consideration; it was shown that there was an increase in the levels of stearic and oleic acid and a decrease in the level of arachidonic acid in pathological tissue with respect to healthy tissue excised from the same patients [143]. In addition, the levels of some polyunsaturated fatty acids were significantly reduced, suggesting an altered lipid metabolism occurring *in vivo* during human bladder tumor-genesis. The only attempt to determine lipid concentrations in urine was made more than 30 years ago in 1985, comparing bladder tumor patients with healthy controls and additionally some patients with bacterial infections. It was shown that there was a marked difference in phospholipid levels compared to fatty acids with 100% specificity and 80% sensitivity. However, macrohematuria or infection can affect the results that subsequently appear similar to the tumor samples [142].

9. Isolated particle

9.1. Exosomes as possible marker

Exosomes are small membrane vesicles particles (30–100 nm) released by the cells into the extracellular environment and play different roles in many physiological situations like the immune response. Exosomes isolated from the urine of patients with muscle-invasive bladder cancer induced epithelial- to mesenchymal transition in urothelial cells [144].

9.2. Analysis of isolated virtosomes from voided urine

Circulating DNA has been isolated using chromatographic separation or by ultracentrifugation. In this way not only cell debris or particles, but also exosomes are eliminated. In the supernatant obtained after ultracentrifugation are present virtosomes that are comprised of newly synthesized DNA, RNA, proteins, and phospholipids and are released from cells in a regulated fashion [145, 146]. In a research made on human lymphocytes in culture, it has been demonstrated that the cells released virtosomes that differ in composition in relation to the stimulation of proliferation made with phytohaemoagglutinin. The virtosomes present in the medium may also be capable of influencing the non-stimulated lymphocytes and *vice versa* [146].

The isolation of virtosomes from voided urine of non-invasive bladder cancer patients has been attempted. The analysis of the material present in the voided urine and from the cell cytoplasm of the control group and the patients are reported in **Table 2**. The nucleic acid content was lower in the patient group, but the difference was not significant and was not confirmed by the cytoplasmic results.

	Urine		**Cytoplasm**	
	Controls	**Patients**	**Controls**	**Patients**
Proteins %	1.5 ± 1.4	1.39 ± 1	0.223 ± 0.19	0.236 ± 0.259
DNA %	0.39 ± 0.31	0.1 ± 0.03	0.143 ± 0.79	0.17 ± 0.029
RNA %	0.09 ± 0.07	0.022 ± 0.007	0.096 ± 0.033	0.056 ± 0.030
PLs %(*)	98.5 ± 1.81	98.35 ± 0.95	99.4 ± 0.32	99.16 ± 0.23

(*) phospholipid.

Table 2. Composition of protein, DNA, RNA, and phospholipid in the voided urine and cell cytoplasm in the control and patient groups.

The values shown in **Table 2** are very different with respect to those obtained from healthy lymphocytes either in the culture medium or in the cytoplasm using the same procedure (**Table 3**), where a much larger proportion of protein and RNA was detected, and only a small proportion of phospholipid [146].

	Medium	**Cytoplasm**
Proteins %	37.91	41.01
DNA %	4.65	3.45
RNA %	53.41	35.09
PLs %(*)	3.94	19.90

(*) phospholipid.

Table 3. Composition of virtosomes isolated from lymphocytes.

The chromatographic analysis of the phospholipids of the voided urine and cell cytoplasm did not show any significant difference between the control and patient groups, unless a small increase in the amount of sphingomyelin in the patient group is considered. However, the most important result was the presence of a large amount of lipids. Preliminary analysis highlighted some differences in the fatty acids that indicated the need for a more in depth analysis (**Table 4**).

Fatty acids presents in the virtosomes					
	Control	%	Low-grade tumor (Ta) %		
Dodecanoate C12:0am==	3.3 μM	1.17	7.9 μM	3.24	↑
Myristate C14:0	22.6 μM	8	15.3 μM	6.28	↓
Pentadecanoate C15:0	27 μM	9.57	13.2 μM	5.4	↓
Palmitate C16:0	98.6 μM	34.9	84.7 μM	34.78	
Heptadecanoate C17:0	16 μM	5.67	11.8 μM	4.84	
Linoleate C18:2n6	18.6 μM	6.59	12 μM	4.92	
Oleate C18:1n9c	20.1 μM	7.12	21.2 μM	8.70	↑
18-methyl nonadecanoate C19:0	1.9 μM	0.67	1 μM	0.41	
Tricosanoic acid C23:0	0.9 μM	0.32	0.3 μM	0.12	↓
Tetracosanoic acid C24:0	2.9 μM	1.02	0.8 μM	0.32	↓
Stearate C18:0	70.2 μM	24.88	75.6 μM	31.04	↑

Table 4. Preliminary analysis that highlighted differences in the fatty acids.

An analysis was also made using chromatographic and mass spectrometric separation by extracting lipids from 20 patients with non-invasive bladder cancer and 20 controls of similar ages (**Figure 2**).

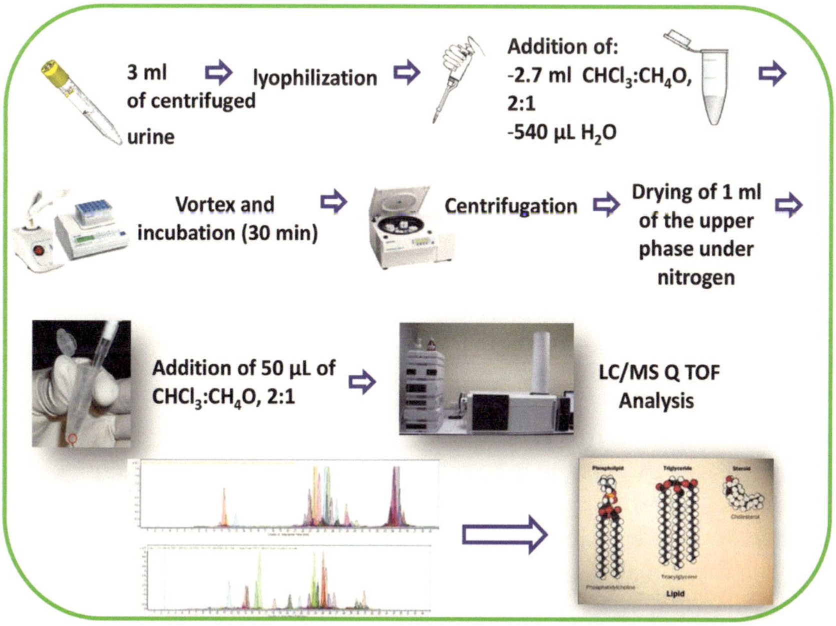

Figure 2. Lipid extraction from urine. Chromatoghraphy and mass-spectrometry of lipids extract from urine [148].

Two hundred and fifty lipids were analyzed and a significant difference was observed, in particular for 25 lipids that appear to be characteristic for the tumor patient. Their identification may offer the possibility of a marker that appears to have sensitivity and a specificity of around 100% (**Figure 3**) [147].

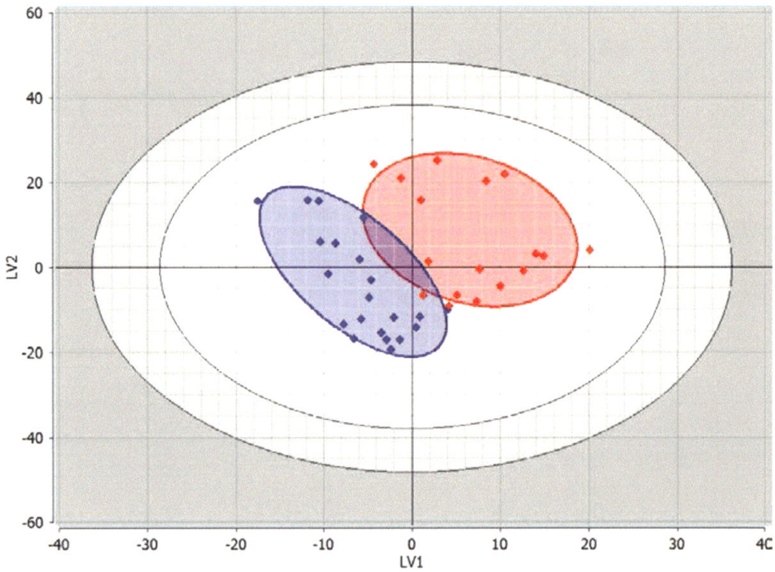

Figure 3. Partial least squares discriminant analysis (PLS-DA). Separation of lipids between patients and heathy controls [146].

10. Conclusions

The numerous publications clearly indicate how important it is to find markers for bladder cancer that may substitute cystoscopy and many efforts were made to find them. The symptoms of the tumor are not always significant and so it is necessary to determine new, specific and sensitive markers for an accurate diagnosis in order to prevent the diffusion of the pathology and to determine the eventual patients at an early stage. This explains the continuous attempts to find good, non-invasive markers, possibly present in the urine. Ideally, they must be cheap so as to allow frequent repeated tests per patient and not technically complex for their use in all laboratories.

The existing markers (such as BTA or NMP22) are not considered sufficiently specific and sensitive for a correct diagnosis and need to be supported by other tests, principally cystoscopy and cytology in which the interpretation depends much on the experience of the analyzer. Therefore, numerous attempts have been made to find other kinds of markers such as DNA mutations, DNA methylation, chromatin modifications, and specific proteins and, more recently, microRNAs present in the urine. To date, all results have been unsatisfactory given the complexity of the analysis and the limited specificity and/or sensitivity. Recently the composition of lipids in the voided urine of patient with non-invasive form and healthy control subjects showed some significant differences thus offering new markers with high sensitivity and specificity. If these preliminary data can be confirmed, a simple and inexpensive test may be produced that is useful for both screening and prognosis.

Acknowledgements

I wish to thank Prof. Peter B. Gahan for revision of manuscript.

Author details

Mariapia Viola-Magni[1*], Samuela Cataldi[2] and Daniela Marocco[1]

*Address all correspondence to: presidente@fondazionepuccinelli.org

1 "Enrico Puccinelli" Onlus Foundation, Perugia, Italy

2 Pharmaceutical Science, University of Perugia, Perugia, Italy

References

[1] American Cancer Society. Key statistics for bladder cancer. How common is bladder cancer? [Internet] Available from: http://www.cancer.org/cancer/bladdercancer/detailedguide/bladder-cancer-key-statistics [Accessed: 2016-11-28]

[2] Kirkali Z, Chan T, Manoharan M, Algaba F, Bush C, Cheng L, Kiemeney L, Kriegmair M, Montironi R, Murphy WM, Sesterhenn IA, Tachibana M, Weider J. Bladder cancer: epidemiology, staging, grading and diagnosis. Urology. 2005; **66**(6A): 4–34. DOI: 10.1016/j.urology.2005.07.062.

[3] Reid LM, Leav I, Kwan PW, Russell P, Merk FB. Characterization of a human, sex steroid-responsive transitional cell carcinoma maintained as a tumor line (R198) in athymic nude mice. Cancer Res. 1984; **44**: 4560–4573.

[4] Yazbek-Hanna M, Whelan P, Jain S. Bladder cancer. Medicine. 2016; **441**: 52–55. DOI: 10.1016/j.mpmed.2015.10.008.

[5] Leppert JT, Shvarts O, Kawaoka K, Lieberman R, Belldegrun AS, Pantuck AJ. Prevention of bladder cancer: a review. Eur Urol. 2006; **49**: 226e34.

[6] Curigliano G, Zhang YJ, Wang LY, Flamini G, Alcini A, Ratto C, Giustacchini M, Alcini E, Cittadini A, Santella RM. Immunohistochemical quantitation of 4-aminobiphenyl-DNA adducts and p53 nuclear overexpressionin T1 bladder cancer of smokers and nonsmokers. Carcinogenesis. 1996; **17**(5): 911–916.

[7] Vineis P, Caporaso N, Tannenbaum SR, Skipper PL, Glogowski J, Bartsch H, Coda M, Talaska G, Kadlubar F. Acetylation phenotype, carcinogen-hemoglobin adducts, and cigarette smoking. Cancer Res. 1990; **50**(10): 3002–3004.

[8] Marcus PM, Hayes RB, Vineis P, Garcia-Closas M, Caporaso NE, Autrup H, Branch RA, Brockmöller J, Ishizaki T, Karakaya AE, Ladero JM, Mommsen S, Okkels H, Romkes M, Roots I, Rothman N. Cigarette smoking, N-acetyltransferase 2 acetylation status, and bladder cancer risk: a case-series meta-analysis of a gene-environment interaction. Cancer Epidemiol Biomarkers. 2000; **9**: 461–467.

[9] Delclos GL, Lerner SP. Occupational risk factors. Scand J Urol Nephrol. 2008; **42**(218): 58–63.

[10] Travis LB, Curtis RE, Glimelius B, Holowaty EJ, Van Leeuwen FE, Lynch CF, Hagenbeek A, Stovall M, Banks PM, Adami J, et al. Bladder and kidney cancer following cyclophosphamide therapy for non-Hodgkin's lymphoma. J Natl Cancer Inst. 1995; **87**: 524–530.

[11] Kaldor JM, Day NE, Kittelmann B, Pettersson F, Langmark F, Pedersen D, Prior P, Neal F, Karjalainen S, Bell J, et al. Bladder tumours following chemotherapy and radiotherapy for ovarian cancer: a case-control study. Int J Cancer. 1995; **63**: 1–6.

[12] Bedwani R, Renganathan E, El Kwhsky F, Braga C, Abu Seif HH, Abul Azm T, Zaki A, Franceschi S, Boffetta P, La Vecchia C. Schistosomiasis and the risk of bladder cancer in Alexandria, Egypt. Br J Cancer. 1998; **77**(7): 1186–1189.

[13] Mustacchi P, Shimkin MD: Cancer of the bladder and infestation with *Schistosoma haematobium*. J Natl Cancer Inst. 1958; **20**: 825–842.

[14] Fletcher O, Easton D, Anderson K, Gilham C, Jay M, Peto J. Lifetime risks of common cancers among retinoblastoma survivors. J Natl Cancer Inst. 2004; **96**: 357–363.

[15] Rambau PF, Chalya PL, Kahima K. Schistosomiasis and urinary bladder cancer in North Western Tanzania: a retrospective review of 185 patients. Infect Agents Cancer.2013; **8**: 19. DOI: 10.1186/1750-9378-8-19.

[16] Shelley MD, Mason MD, Kynaston H. Intravesical therapy for superficial bladder cancer: a systematic review of randomised trials and meta-analyses. Cancer Treat Rev. 2010; **36**: 95–205.

[17] Proctor I, Kai Stoeber K, Williams GH. Biomarkers in bladder cancer. Histopathology. 2010; **57**: 1–13. DOI: 10.1111/j.1365-2559.2010.03592.x.

[18] Darwiche F, Parekh DJ, Gonzalgo ML. Biomarkers for non-muscle invasive bladder cancer: current tests and future promise. Indian J Urol. 2015; **31**(4): 273–282. DOI: 10.1155/2016/8205836.

[19] Mossanen M, Gore JL. The burden of bladder cancer care: direct and indirect costs. Curr Opin Urol. 2014; **24**(5): 487–491. DOI: 10.1097/MOU.0000000000000078.

[20] Chao D, Freedland SJ, Pantuck AJ, Zisman A, Belldegrun AS. Bladder cancer 2000: molecular markers for the diagnosis of transitional cell carcinoma. Rev Urol. 2001; **3**(2): 85–93.

[21] Murphy WM, Soloway MS, Jukkola AF, Crabtree WN, Ford KS. Urinary cytology and bladder cancer. The cellular features of transitional cell neoplasms. Cancer. 1984; **53**: 1555–1565.

[22] Goodison S, Rosser CJ, Urquidi V. Bladder cancer detection and monitoring: assessment of urine- and blood-based marker tests. Mol Diagn Ther. 2013; **17**(2): 71–84. DOI: 10.1007/s40291-013-0023-x.

[23] D'Costa JJ, Goldsmith JC, Wilson JS, Bryan RT, Ward DG. A systematic review of the diagnostic and prognostic value of urinary protein biomarkers in urothelial bladder cancer. Bladder Cancer. 2016; **2**(3): 301–317.

[24] Urquidi V, Rosser CJ, Goodison S. Molecular diagnostic trends in urological cancer: biomarkers for non-invasive diagnosis. Curr Med Chem. 2012; **19**(22): 3653–3663.

[25] Gutiérrez Baños JL, del Henar Rebollo Rodrigo M, Antolín Juárez FM, García BM. Usefulness of the BTA STAT test for the diagnosis of bladder cancer. Urology. 2001; **57**(4): 685–689.

[26] Menendez V, Filella X, Alcover JA, Molina R, Mallafre JM, Ballesta AM, Talbot-Wright R. Usefulness of urinary matrix protein 22 (NMP22) as a marker for transitional cell carcinoma of the bladder. Anticancer Res. 2000; **20**: 1169–1172.

[27] Sánchez-Carbayo M, Herrero E, Megías J, Mira A, Soria F. Evaluation of nuclear matrix protein 22 as a tumor marker in the detection of transitional cell carcinoma of the bladder. Br J Urol Int. 1999; **84**: 706–713.

[28] Soloway MS, Briggman V, Carpinito GA, Chodak GW, Church PA, Lamm DL, Lange P, Messing E, Pasciak RM, Reservitz GB, Rukstalis DB, Sarosdy MF, Stadler WM, Thiel RP, Hayden CL. Use of a new tumor marker, urinary NMP22, in the detection of occult or rapidly recurring transitional cell carcinoma of the urinary tract following surgical treatment. J Urol. 1996; **156**: 363–367.

[29] Getzenberg RH, Konety BR, Oeler TA. Bladder cancer-associated nuclear matrix proteins. Cancer Res. 1996; **56**(7): 1690–1694.

[30] Santoni M, Catanzariti F, Minardi D, Burattini L, Nabissi M, Muzzonigro G, Cascinu S, Santoni G. Pathogenic and diagnostic potential of BLCA-1 and BLCA-4 nuclear proteins in urothelial cell carcinoma of human bladder. Adv Urol. 2012; **2012**: 397412. DOI: 10.1155/2012/397412.

[31] Yang J, Li Y, Khoury T, Alrawi S, Goodrich DW, Tan D. Relationships of hHpr1/p84/Thoc1 expression to clinicopathologic characteristics and prognosis in non-small cell lung cancer. Ann Clin Lab Sci. 2008; **38**(2): 105–112.

[32] Van Le TS, Myers J, Konety BR, Barder T, Getzenberg RH. Functional characterization of the bladder cancer marker, BLCA-4. Clin Cancer Res. 2004; **10**(4): 1384-1391

[33] Mady EA. Cytokeratins as serum markers in egyptian bladder cancer. A comparison of CYFRA 21-1, TPA and TPS. Int J Biol Marker. 2001; **16**(2): 130–135.

[34] Nisman B, Barak V, Shapiro A, Golijanin D, Peretz T, Pode D. Evaluation of urine CYFRA 21-1 for the detection of primary and recurrent bladder carcinoma. Cancer. 2002; **94**(11): 2914–2922.

[35] Sánchez-Carbayo M, Herrero E, Megías J, Mira A, Soria F. Initial evaluation of the new urinary bladder cancer rapid test in the detection of transitional cell carcinoma of the bladder. Urology. 1999; **54**: 656–661.

[36] Mian C, Lodde M, Haitel A, Vigl EE, Marberger M, Pycha A. Comparison of two qualitative assays, the UBC rapid test and the BTA STAT test, in the diagnosis of urothelial cell carcinoma of the bladder. Urology. 2000; **56**(2): 228–231.

[37] Babjuk M, Soukup V, Pesl M, Kostírová M, Drncová E, Smolová H, Szakacsová M, Getzenberg R, Pavlík I, Dvorácek J. Urinary cytology and quantitative BTA and UBC tests in surveillance of patients with pTapT1 bladder urothelial carcinoma. Urology. 2008; **71**(4): 718–722. DOI: 10.1016/j.urology.2007.12.021.

[38] Dittadi R, Barioli P, Gion M, Gianneo E. Standardization of assay for cytokeratin-related tumor marker CYFRA 21.1 in urine samples. Clin Chem. 1996; **42**: 1634–1638.

[39] Altieri DC. Survivin, versatile modulation of cell division and apoptosis in cancer. Oncogene. 2003; **22**(53): 8581.

[40] Lokeshwar VB, Habuchi T, Grossman HB, Murphy WM, Hautmann SH, Hemstreet GP 3rd, Bono AV, Getzenberg RH, Goebell P, Schmitz-Dräger BJ, Schalken JA, Fradet Y, Marberger M, Messing E, Droller MJ. Bladder tumor markers beyond cytology: international consensus panel on bladder tumor markers. Urology. 2005; **66**: 35–63.

[41] Shariat SF, Casella R, Khoddami SM, Hernandez G, Sulser T, Gasser TC, Lerner SP. Urine detection of survivin is a sensitive marker for the noninvasive diagnosis of bladder cancer. J Urol. 2004; **171**(2 Pt 1): 626–630.

[42] Greene KL, Berry A, Konety BR. Diagnostic utility of the ImmunoCyt/uCyt+ test in bladder cancer. Rev Urol. 2006; **8**: 190–197.

[43] Leivo MZ, Elson PJ, Tacha DE, Delahunt B, Hansel DE. A combination of p40, GATA-3 and uroplakin II shows utility in the diagnosis and prognosis of muscle-invasive urothelial carcinoma. Pathology. 2016; **48**(6): 543–549. DOI: 10.1016/j.pathol.2016.05.008.

[44] Dimashkieh H, Wolff DJ, Smith TM, Houser PM, Nietert PJ, Yang J. Evaluation of urovysion and cytology for bladder cancer detection: a study of 1835 paired urine samples with clinical and histologic correlation. Cancer Cytopathol. 2013; **121**: 591–597.

[45] Gilbert SM, Veltri RW, Sawczuk A, Shabsigh A, Knowles DR, Bright S, O'Dowd GJ, Olsson CA, Benson MC, Sawczuk IS. Evaluation of DD23 as a marker for detection of recurrent transitional cell carcinoma of the bladder in patients with a history of bladder cancer. Urology. 2003; **61**(3): 539–543.

[46] Bonner RB, Liebert M, Hurst RE, Grossman HB, Bane BL, Hemstreet GP 3rd. Characterization of the DD23 tumor-associated antigen for bladder cancer detection and recurrence monitoring. Marker network for bladder cancer. Cancer Epidemiol Biomarkers Prev. 1996; **5**(12): 971–978.

[47] Sawczuk IS, Pickens CL, Vasa UR, Ralph DA, Norris KA, Miller MC, Ng AY, Grossman HB, Veltri RW. DD23 Biomarker: a prospective clinical assessment in routine urinary cytology specimens from patients being monitored for TCC. Urol Oncol. 2002; **7**(5): 185–190.

[48] Murphy WM. Current status of urinary cytology in the evaluation of bladder neoplasms. Human Path. 1990; **21**(9): 886–896.

[49] Badalament RA, Hermansen DK, Kimmel M, Gay H, Herr HW, Fair WR, Whitmore WF Jr, Melamed MR. The sensitivity of bladder wash flow cytometry, bladder wash cytology, and voided cytology in the detection of bladder carcinoma. Cancer. 1987; **60**(7): 1423–1427.

[50] Slaton JW, Dinney CPN, Veltri RW, Miller MC, Liebert M, O'Dowd GJ, Grossman HB. Deoxyribonucleic acid ploidy enhances the cytological prediction of recurrent transitional cell carcinoma of the bladder. J Urol. 1997; **158**(3 Pt 1): 806–811.

[51] Fradet Y, Cordon CC. Critical appraisal of tumor markers in bladder cancer. Sem in Urol.1993; **11**(3): 145–153.

[52] Burchardt M, Burchardt T, Shabsigh A, De La Taille A, Benson MC, Sawczuk I. Current concepts in biomarker technology for bladder cancers. Clin Chem. 2000; **46**(5): 595–605.

[53] Koss LG, editor. Diagnostic Cytology and its Histologic Bases. vol. 2. Lippincott: Philadelphia; 1979.

[54] Murphy WM. Current status of urinary cytology in the evaluation of bladder neoplasms. Human Pathlo. 1990; **21**(9): 886–896.

[55] Birkenkamp-Demtröder K, Nordentoft I, Christensen E, Høyer S, Reinert T, Vang S, Borre M, Agerbæk M, Jensen JB, Ørntoft TF, Dyrskjøt L. Genomic alterations in liquid biopsies from patients with bladder cancer. Eur Urol. 2016; **70**(1): 75–82. DOI: 10.1016/j.eururo.2016.01.007.

[56] Cancer Genome Atlas Research Network. Comprehensive molecular characterization of urothelial bladder carcinoma. Nature. 2014; **507**(7492): 315–322. DOI: 10.1038/naturc12965.

[57] Frantzi M, Makridakis M, Vlahou A. Biomarkers for bladder cancer aggressiveness. Curr Opin Urol. 2012; **22**(5): 390–396. DOI: 10.1097/MOU.0b013e328356ad0e.

[58] Critelli R, Fasanelli F, Oderda M, Polidoro S, Assumma MB, Viberti C, Preto M, Gontero P, Cucchiarale G, Lurkin I, Zwarthoff EC, Vineis P, Sacerdote C, Matullo G, Naccarati A. Detection of multiple mutations in urinary exfoliated cells from male bladder cancer patients at diagnosis and during follow-up. Oncotarget. 2016; **7**(41):67435–67448. DOI: 10.18632/oncotarget.11883.

[59] Wu P, Cao Z, Wu S. New progress of epigenetic biomarkers in urological cancer. Dis Markers. 2016; **2016**: 9864047. DOI: 10.1155/2016/9864047.

[60] Kim EJ, Kim YJ, Jeong P, Ha YS, Bae SC, Kim WJ. Methylation of the RUNX3 promoter as a potential prognostic marker for bladder tumor. J Urol. 2008; **180**(3): 1141–1145.

[61] Roperch JP, Grandchamp B, Desgrandchamps F, Mongiat-Artus P, Ravery V, Ouzaid I, Roupret M, Phe V, Ciofu C, Tubach F, Cussenot O, Incitti R. Promoter hypermethylation of HS3ST2, SEPTIN9 and SLIT2 combined with FGFR3 mutations as a sensitive/specific urinary assay for diagnosis and surveillance in patients with low or high-risk non-muscle-invasive bladder cancer. BMC Cancer. 2016; **16**(1): 704. DOI: 10.1186/s12885-016-2748-5.

[62] Chen F, Huang T,Ren Y, Wei J, Lou Z, Wang X,Fan X, Chen Y, Weng G, Yao X. Clinical significance of CDH13 promoter methylation as a biomarker for bladder cancer: a meta-analysis. BMC Urol. 2016; **16**(1): 52. DOI: 10.1186/s12894-016-0171-5.

[63] Takeuchi T, Ohtsuki Y. Recent progress in t-cadherin (cdh13, h-cadherin) research. J Histol Histopathol. 2001; **16**: 1287–1293.

[64] Andreeva AV, Kutuzov MA. Cadherin 13 in cancer. Genes Chromosomes Cancer. 2010; **49**(9): 775–790.

[65] Mao L, Schoenberg MP, Scicchitano M, Erozan YS, Merlo A, Schwab D, Sidransky D. Molecular detection of primary bladder cancer by microsatellite analysis. Science. 1996; **271**(5249): 659–662.

[66] Mao L, Lee DJ, Tockman MS, Erozan YS, Askin F, Sidransky D. Microsatellite alterations as clonal markers for the detection of human cancer. Proc Natl Acad Sci U S A. 1994; **91**: 9871–9875.

[67] Christensen M, Jensen MA, Wolf H, Orntoft TF. Pronounced microsatellite instability in transitional cell carcinomas from young patients with bladder cancer. Int J Cancer. 1998; **79**: 396–401.

[68] Berger AP, Parson W, Stenzl A, Steiner H, Bartsch G, Klocker H. Microsatellite alterations in human bladder cancer: detection of tumor cells in urine sediment and tumor tissue. Eur Urol. 2002; **41**: 53–539.

[69] Catto JW, Azzouzi AR, Amira N, Rehman I, Feeley KM, Cross SS, Fromont G, Sibony M, Hamdy FC, Cussenot O, Meuth M. Distinct patterns of microsatellite instability are seen in tumours of the urinary tract. Oncogene. 2003; **22**: 8699–8706.

[70] Saidi S, Popov Z, Stavridis S, Panov S. Alterations of microsatellite loci GSN and D18S51 in urinary bladder cancer. Hippokratia. 2015; **19**(3): 200–204.

[71] Bonnal C, Ravery V, Toublanc M, Bertrand G, Boccon-Gibod L, Hénin D, Grandchamp B. Absence of microsatellite instability in transitional cell carcinoma of the bladder. Urology. 2000; **55**: 287–291.

[72] Vaish M, Mandhani A, Mittal RD, Mittal B. Microsatellite instability as prognostic marker in bladder tumors: a clinical significance. BMC Urol. 2005; **5**: 2.

[73] Li QQ, Hao JJ, Zhang Z, Hsu I, Liu Y, Tao Z, Lewi K, Metwalli AR, Agarwal PK. Histone deacetylase inhibitor-induced cell death in bladder cancer is associated with chromatin modification and modifying protein expression: a proteomic approach. Int J Oncol. 2016; **48**(6): 2591–607. DOI: 10.3892/ijo.2016.3478.

[74] Varticovski L, Kim S, Nickerson ML, Thompson B, Lao Q, Grøntved L, Baek S, Sung MH, Theodorescu D, Dean M, Hager GL. Abstract 4783: novel molecular markers of bladder cancer progression identified by global chromatin profiling. Cancer Res. 2015; **75**(15 Suppl): 4783–4783. DOI: 10.1158/1538-7445.AM2015-4783.

[75] Hassler MR, Egger G. Epigenomics of cancer – emerging new concepts. Biochimie. 2012; **94**(11): 2219–2230. DOI: 10.1016/j.biochi.2012.05.007.

[76] Marks P, Rifkind RA, Richon VM, Breslow R, Miller T, Kelly WK. Histone deacetylases and cancer: Causes and therapies. Nat Rev Cancer. 2001; **1**: 194–202.

[77] Xu WS, Parmigiani RB, Marks PA. Histone deacetylase inhibitors: molecular mechanisms of action. Oncogene. 2007; **26**(37): 5541–5552.

[78] Marks PA, Xu WS. Histone deacetylase inhibitors: potential in cancer therapy. J Cell Biochem. 2009; **107**: 600–608.

[79] Schrump DS. Cytotoxicity mediated by histone deacetylase inhibitors in cancer cells: mechanisms and potential clinical implications. Clin Cancer Res. 2009; **15**: 3947–3957.

[80] Nakagawa M, Oda Y, Eguchi T, Aishima S, Yao T, Hosoi F, Basaki Y, Ono M, Kuwano M, Tanaka M, Tsuneyoshi M. Expression profile of class I histone deacetylases in human cancer tissues. Oncol Rep. 2007; **18**: 769–774.

[81] Zhang Z, Yamashita H, Toyama T, Sugiura H, Ando Y, Mita K, Hamaguchi M, Hara Y, Kobayashi S, Iwase H. Quantitation of HDAC1 mRNA expression in invasive carcinoma of the breast. Breast Cancer Res Treat. 2005; **94**: 11–16.

[82] Marquard L, Poulsen CB, Gjerdrum LM, de Nully Brown P, Christensen IJ, Jensen PB, Sehested M, Johansen P, Ralfkiaer E. Histone deacetylase 1, 2, 6 and acetylated histone H4 in B- and T-cell lymphomas. Histopathology. 2009; **54**: 688–698.

[83] Witt O, Deubzer HE, Milde T, Oehme I. HDAC family: What are the cancer relevant targets. Cancer Lett. 2009; **277**: 8–21.

[84] Mezzasoma L, Antognelli C, Del Buono C, Stracci F, Cottini E, Cochetti G, Talesa VN, Mearini E. Expression and biological-clinical significance of hTR, hTERT and CKS2 in washing fluids of patients with bladder cancer. BMC Urology 2010; **10**: 17. DOI: 10.1186/1471-2490-10-17.

[85] Zakian VA. Life and cancer without telomerase. Cell. 1997; **91**(1): 1–3.

[86] Halling KC, King W, Sokolova IA, Karnes RJ, Meyer RG, Powell EL, Sebo TJ, Cheville JC, Clayton AC, Krajnik KL, Ebert TA, Nelson RE, Burkhardt HM, Ramakumar S, Stewart CS, Pankratz VS, Lieber MM, Blute ML, Zincke H, Seelig SA, Jenkins RB, O'Kane DJ. A comparison of BTA STAT, hemoglobin dipstick, telomerase and Vysis UroVysion assays for the detection of urothelial carcinoma in urine. J Urol. 2002; **167**(5): 2001–2006.

[87] Keesee SK, Briggman JV, Thill G, Wu YJ. Utilization of nuclear matrix proteins for cancer diagnosis. Crit Rev Eukaryot Gene Expr. 1996; **6**(2–3): 189–214.

[88] Ulaner GA, Hu JF, Vu TH, Giudice LC, Hoffman AR. Telomerase activity in human development is regulated by human telomerase reverse transcriptase (hTERT) transcription and by alternate splicing of hTERT transcripts. Cancer Res. 1998; **58**(18): 4168–4172.

[89] Kavaler E, Landman J, Chang Y,Yongli Chang BA, Droller MJ, Brian C. Detecting human bladder carcinoma cells in voided urine samples by assaying for the presence of telomerase activity. Cancer. 1998; **82**: 708–714.

[90] Lee DH, Yang SC, Hong SJ, Chung BH, Kim IY. Telomerase; a potential marker of bladder transitional cell carcinoma in bladder washes. Clin Cancer Res. 1998; **4**(3): 535–538.

[91] Yoshida K, Sugino T, Tahara H, Woodman A, Bolodeoku J, Nargund V, Fellows G, Goodison S, Tahara E, Tarin D. Detection of telomerase activity in exfoliated cells in urine from patients with bladder cancer. Cancer. 1997; **79**(2): 362–369.

[92] Dalbagni G, Han W, Zhang ZF, Cordon-Cardo C, Saigo P, Fair WR, Herr H, Kim N, Moore MA. Evaluation of the telomeric repeat amplification protocol (TRAP) assay for telomerase as a diagnostic modality in recurrent bladder cancer. Clin Cancer Res. 1997; **3**(9): 1593–1598.

[93] Wu XX, Kakehi Y, Takahashi T, Habuchi T, Ogawa O. Telomerase activity in urine after transurethral resection of superficial bladder cancer and early recurrence. Int J Urol. 2000; **7**(6): 210–217.

[94] Bhuiyan J, Akhter J, O'Kane DJ. Performance characteristics of multiple urinary tumor markers and sample collection techniques in the detection of transitional cell carcinoma of the bladder. Clin Chim Acta. 2003; **331**(1–2): 69–77.

[95] Bialkowska-Hobrzanska H, Bowles L, Bukala B, Joseph MG, Fletcher R, Razvi H. Comparison of human telomerase reverse transcriptase messenger RNA and telomerase activity as urine markers for diagnosis of bladder carcinoma. Mol Diagn. 2000; **5**(4): 267–277.

[96] De Kok JB, Schalken JA, Aalders TW, Ruers TJ, Willems HL, Swinkels DW. Quantitative measurement of telomerase reverse transcriptase (hTERT) mRNA in urothelial cell carcinomas. Int J Cancer. 2000; **87**(2): 217–220.

[97] Hanke M, Kausch I, Dahmen G, Jocham D, Warnecke JM. Detailed technical. Analysis of urine RNA-based tumor diagnostics reveals ETS2/urokinase plasminogen activator to be a novel marker for bladder cancer. Clin Chem. 2007; **53**(12): 2070–2077. DOI: 10.1373/clinchem.2007.091363.

[98] Buggy Y, Maguire TM, McDermott E, Hill AD, O'Higgins N, Duffy MJ. Ets2 transcription factor in normal and neoplastic human breast tissue. Eur J Cancer. 2006; **42**: 485–491.

[99] Duffy MJ, Duggan C. The urokinase plasminogen activator system: a rich source of tumour markers for the individualised management of patients with cancer. Clin Biochem. 2004; **37**: 541–548.

[100] Casella R, Shariat SF, Monoski MA, Lerner SP. Urinary levels of urokinase-type plasminogen activator and its receptor in the detection of bladder carcinoma. Cancer. 2002; **95**: 2494–2499.

[101] Bhuvarahamurthy V, Schroeder J, Denkert C, Kristiansen G, Schnorr D, Loening SA, et al. In situ gene expression of urokinase-type plasminogen activator and its receptor in transitional cell carcinoma of the human bladder. Oncol Rep. 2004; **12**: 909–913.

[102] Hedegaard, Jakob et al. Comprehensive Transcriptional Analysis of Early-Stage Urothelial Carcinoma. Cancer Cell. 2016; **30**(1): 27–43

[103] Kim D, Pertea G, Trapnell C, Pimentel H, Kelley R, Salzberg SL. TopHat2: accurate alignment of transcriptomes in the presence of insertions, deletions and gene fusions. Genome Biol. 2013; **14**(4): R36. DOI: 10.1186/gb-2013-14-4-r36.

[104] Trapnell C, Williams BA, Pertea G, Mortazavi A, Kwan G, van Baren MJ, Salzberg SL, Wold BJ, Pachter L. Transcript assembly and quantification by RNA-Seq reveals unannotated transcripts and isoform switching during cell differentiation. Nat Biotechnol. 2010; **28**(5): 511–515. DOI: 10.1038/nbt.1621.

[105] Sjödahl G, Lauss M, Lövgren K, Chebil G, Gudjonsson S, Veerla S, Patschan O, Aine M, Fernö M, Ringnér M, Månsson W, Liedberg F, Lindgren D, Höglund M. A molecular taxonomy for urothelial carcinoma. Clin Cancer Res. 2012; **18**(12): 3377–3386. DOI: 10.1158/1078-0432.CCR-12-0077-T.

[106] Dyrskjøt L, Zieger K, Real FX, Malats N, Carrato A, Hurst C, Kotwal S, Knowles M, Malmström PU, de la Torre M, Wester K, Allory Y, Vordos D, Caillault A, Radvanyi F, Hein AM, Jensen JL, Jensen KM, Marcussen N, Orntoft TF. Gene expression signatures predict outcome in non-muscle-invasive bladder carcinoma: a multicenter validation study. Clin Cancer Res. 2007; **13**(12): 3545–3551.

[107] Patel N, Sauter ER. Body fluid micro(mi)RNAs as biomarkers for human cancer. J Nucleic Acids Investig. 2011; **2**: e1. DOI: 10.4081/jnai.2011.e1.

[108] Enokida H, Yoshino H, Matsushita R, Nakagawa M. The role of microRNAs in bladder cancer. Investig Clin Urol. 2016; **57**(Suppl 1): S60–S76. DOI: 10.4111/icu.2016.57.S1.S60.

[109] Lee H, Jun SY, Lee YS, Lee HJ, Lee WS, Park CS. Expression of miRNAs and ZEB1 and ZEB2 correlates with histopathological grade in papillary urothelial tumors of the urinary bladder. Virchows Arch. 2014; **464**(2): 213–220. DOI: 10.1007/s00428-013-1518-x.

[110] Croce CM. Causes and consequences of microRNA dysregulation in cancer. Nat Rev Genet. 2009; 10(10): 704–714.

[111] Yamada Y, Enokida H, Kojima S, Kawakami K, Chiyomaru T, Tatarano S, Yoshino H, Kawahara K, Nishiyama K, Seki N, Nakagawa M. MiR-96 and miR-183 detection in urine serve as potential tumor markers of urothelial carcinoma: correlation with stage and grade, and comparison with urinary cytology. Cancer Sci. 2011; **102**(3): 522–529. DOI: 10.1111/j.1349-7006.2010.01816.x.

[112] Shimizu T, Suzuki H, Nojima M, Kitamura H, Yamamoto E, Maruyama R, Ashida M, Hatahira T, Kai M, Masumori N, Tokino T, Imai K, Tsukamoto T, Toyota M. Methylation of a panel of microRNA genes is a novel biomarker for detection of bladder cancer. Eur Urol. 2013; **63**(6): 1091–1100. DOI: 10.1016/j.eururo.2012.11.030.

[113] Jiang X, Du L, Wang L, Li J, Liu Y, Zheng G, Qu A, Zhang X, Pan H, Yang Y, Wang C. Serum microRNA expression signatures identified from genome-wide microRNA profiling serve as novel noninvasive biomarkers for diagnosis and recurrence of bladder cancer. Int J Cancer. 2015; **136**: 854–862.

[114] Kim SM, Kang HW, Kim WT, Kim YJ, Yun SJ, Lee SC, Kim WJ. Cell-free microRNA-214 from urine as a biomarker for non-muscle-invasive bladder cancer. Korean J Urol. 2013; **54**: 791–796.

[115] Zhang X, Zhang Y, Liu X, Fang A, Li P, Li Z, Liu T, Yang Y, Du L, Wang C. MicroRNA-203 is a prognostic indicator in bladder cancer and enhances chemosensitivity to cisplatin via apoptosis by targeting Bcl-w and survivin. PLoS One. 2015; **10**: e0143441.

[116] Li CY, Li HJ, Zhang T, Gao HS, Chang JW, Men XL, et al. Significance of apolipoprotein A1 as biomarker for early diagnosis and classification of bladder urothelial carcinoma. Zhonghua Lao Dong Wei Sheng Zhi Ye Bing Za Zhi. 2013; **31**(4): 266–270.

[117] Li LY, Yang M, Zhang HB, Su XK, Xu WF, Chen Y, Shen ZJ, Gao X. Urinary fibronectin as a predictor of a residual tumour load after transurethral resection of bladder transitional cell carcinoma. BJU Int. 2008; **102**(5): 566–571.

[118] Mutlu N, Turkeri L, Emerk K. Analytical and clinical evaluation of a new urinary tumor marker: bladder tumor fibronectin in diagnosis and follow-up of bladder cancer. Clin Chem Lab Med. 2003; **41**(8): 1069–1074.

[119] Alías-Melgar A, Neave-Sánchez E, Suárez-Cuenca JA, Morales-Covarrubias J. Association of urine oncofetal fibronectin levels with urology's most common disorders. Ann Clin Lab Sci. 2013; **43**(4): 420–423.

[120] Hazzaa S, Elashry O, Afifi I. Clusterin as a diagnostic and prognostic marker for transitional cell carcinoma of the bladder. Pathol Oncol Res. 2010; **16**(1): 101–109.

[121] Jenne D, Tschopp J. Clusterin: the intriguing guises of a widely expressed glycoprotein. Trends Biochem Sci. 1992; **17**(4): 154–159.

[122] Tilki D, Singer BB, Shariat SF, Behrend A, Fernando M, Irmak S, Buchner A, Hooper AT, Stief CG, Reich O, Ergün S. CEACAM A novel urinary marker for bladder cancer detection. Eur Urol. 2010; **57**(4): 648–654.

[123] Ebbing J, Mathia S, Seibert FS, Pagonas N, Bauer F, Erber B, Günzel K, Kilic E, Kempkensteffen C, Miller K, Bachmann A, Rosenberger C, Zidek W, Westhoff TH. Urinary calprotectin: a new diagnostic marker in urothelial carcinoma of the bladder. World J Urol. 2014; **32**(6): 1485–1492.

[124] Minami S, Sato Y, Matsumoto T, Kageyama T, Kawashima Y, Yoshio K, Ishii J, Matsumoto K, Nagashio R, Okayasu I. Proteomic study of sera from patients with bladder cancer: usefulness of S100A8 and S100A9 proteins. Cancer Genomics Proteomics. 2010; **7**(4): 181–189.

[125] Tolson JP, Flad T, Gnau V, Dihazi H, Hennenlotter J, Beck A, Mueller GA, Kuczyk M, Mueller CA. Differential detection of S100A8 in transitional cell carcinoma of the bladder by pair wise tissue proteomic and immunohistochemical analysis. Proteomics. 2006; **6**(2): 697–708.

[126] Bhagirath D, Abrol N, Khan R, Sharma M, Seth A, Sharma A. Expression of CD147, BIGH3 and Stathmin and their potential role as diagnostic marker in patients with urothelial carcinoma of the bladder. Clin Chim Acta. 2012; **413**(19–20): 1641–1646.

[127] Hemdan T, Lindén M, Lind SB, Namuduri AV, Sjöstedt E, de Ståhl TD, Asplund A, Malmström PU, Segersten U. The prognostic value and therapeutic target role of stathmin-1 in urinary bladder cancer. Br J Cancer. 2014; **111**(6): 1180–1187. DOI: 10.1038/bjc.2014.427.

[128] Afonso J, Longatto-Filho A, Baltazar F, Sousa N, Costa FE, Morais A, Amaro T, Lopes C, Santos LL. CD147 overexpression allows an accurate discrimination of bladder cancer patients' prognosis. Eur J Surg Oncol. 2011; **37**(9): 811–817.

[129] Lee H, Choi S, Ro J. Overexpression of DJ-1 and HSP90α, and loss of PTEN associated with invasive urothelial carcinoma of urinary bladder: Possible prognostic markers. Oncol Lett. 2012; **3**(3): 507–512.

[130] D'Costa JJ, Goldsmith JC, Wilson JS, Bryan RT, Ward DG. A systematic review of the diagnostic and prognostic value of urinary protein biomarkers in urothelial bladder cancer. Bl Cancer. 2016; **2**(3): 301–317. DOI: 10.3233/BLC-160054.

[131] Chen CL, Lin TS, Tsai CH, Wu CC, Chung T, Chien KY, Wu M, Chang YS, Yu JS, Chen YT. Identification of potential bladder cancer markers in urine by abundant-protein depletion coupled with quantitative proteomics. J Proteomics. 2013; **85**: 28–43. DOI: 10.1016/j.jprot.2013.04.024.

[132] Kumar P, Nandi S, Tan TZ, Ler SG, Chia KS, Lim WY, Bütow Z, Vordos D, De la Taille A, Al-Haddawi M, Raida M, Beyer B, Ricci E, Colombel M, Chong TW, Chiong E, Soo R, Park MK, Ha HK, Gunaratne J, Thiery JP. Highly sensitive and specific novel biomarkers for the diagnosis of transitional bladder carcinoma. Oncotarget. 2015; **6**(15): 13539–13549.

[133] Orenes-Piñero E, Cortón M, González-Peramato P, Algaba F, Casal I, Serrano A, Sánchez-Carbayo M.Searching urinary tumor markers for bladder cancer using a two-dimensional differential gel electrophoresis (2D-DIGE) approach. J Proteome Res. 2007; **6**: 4440–4448.

[134] Chen LM, Chang M, Dai Y, Chai KX, Dyrskjøt L, Sanchez-Carbayo M, Szarvas T, Zwarthoff EC, Lokeshwar V, Jeronimo C, Parker AS, Ross S, Borre M, Orntoft TF, Jaeger T, Beukers W, Lopez LE, Henrique R, Young PR, Urquidi V, Goodison S, Rosser CJ. External validation of a multiplex urinary protein panel for the detection of bladder cancer in a multicenter cohort. Cancer Epidemiol Biomarkers Prev. 2014; **23**(9): 1804–1812. DOI: 10.1158/1055-9965.

[135] Eissa S, Ali-Labib R, Swellam M, Bassiony M, Tash F, El-Zayat T. Noninvasive diagnosis of bladder cancer by detection of matrix metalloproteinases (MMP-2 and MMP-9) and their inhibitor (TIMP-2) in urine. Eur Urol. 2007; **52**(5): 1388–1396.

[136] Eissa S, Labib RA, Mourad MS, Kamel K, El-Ahmady O. Comparison of telomerase activity and matrix metalloproteinase-9 in voided urine and bladder wash samples as a useful diagnostic tool for bladder cancer. Eur Urol. 2003; **44**(6): 687–694.

[137] El-Sharkawi F, El Sabah M, Hassan Z, Khaled H. The biochemical value of urinary metalloproteinases 3 and 9 in diagnosis and prognosis of bladder cancer in Egypt. J Biomed Sci. 2014; **21**(1): 72. DOI: 10.1186/s12929-014-0072-4.

[138] Fernández CA, Wszolek MF, Loughlin KR, Libertino JA, Summerhayes IC, Shuber AP. A novel approach to using matrix metalloproteinases for bladder cancer. J Urol. 2009; **182**(5): 2188–2194.

[139] Mohammed MA, Seleim MF, Abdalla MS, Sharada HM, Abdel WAH. Urinary high molecular weight matrix metalloproteinases as non-invasive biomarker for detection of bladder cancer. BMC Urol. 2013; **13**(1):25. DOI: 10.1186/1471-2490-13-25.

[140] Rosser CJ, Dai Y, Miyake M, Zhang G, Goodison S. Simultaneous multi-analyte urinary protein assay for bladder cancer detection. BMC Biotechnol. 2014; **14**(1): 24. DOI: 10.1186/1472-6750-14-24

[141] Urquidi V, Kim J, Chang M, Dai Y, Rosser CJ, Goodison S. CCL18 in a multiplex urine-based assay for the detection of bladder cancer. PLoS One. 2012; **7**(5):e37797. DOI: 10.1371/journal.pone.0037797

[142] Llopis B, Gallego J, Cruz M, Martínez M, Mompó JA, Jiménez JF. Urinary lipids in vesical carcinoma: a new biological marker. Preliminary study. Eur Urol. 1985; **11**(2): 121–126.

[143] Miryaghoubzadeh J, Darabi M, Madaen K, Shaaker M, Mehdizadeh A, Hajihosseini R. Tissue fatty acid composition in human urothelial carcinoma. Br J Biomed Sci. 2013; **70**(1): 1–5.

[144] Nagata M, Muto S, Horie S. Molecular biomarkers in bladder cancer: novel potential indicators of prognosis and treatment outcomes. Dis Markers. 2016; **2016**: 8205836. DOI: 10.1155/2016/8205836.

[145] Gahan PB, Stroun M. The virtosome-a novel cytosolic informative entity and intercellular messenger. Cell Biochem Funct. 2010; **28**(7): 529–538. DOI: 10.1002/cbf.1690.

[146] Cataldi S, Viola-Magni M. Components of the cytosolic and released virtosomes from stimulated and non-stimulated human lymphocytes. Biochemistry and Biophysics Reports. 2016; **6**: 236–241. DOI: 10.1016/j.bbrep.2016.04.006.

[147] Cruciani G, Cataldi S, Costantini E, Di Veroli A, Goracci L, Pellegrino R, Sidoni A, Viola-Magni M. In preparation.

[148] Bang DY, Byeon SK, Moon MH. Method by Rapid and simple extraction of lipids from blood plasma and urine for liquid chromatography-tandem mass spectrometry. J Chromatogr A. 2014; **1331**: 19–26.

Section 2

Muscle-Invasive Bladder Cancer and Radical Cystectomy

Chapter 5

Lymphadenectomy in Muscle Invasive Bladder Cancer

Mustafa Ozan Horsanali and Kutan Ozer

Additional information is available at the end of the chapter

http://dx.doi.org/10.5772/67443

Abstract

Bladder cancer is the second most common genitourinary malignancy with urothelial cancer comprising nearly 90% of primary bladder tumors. Urothelial carcinoma of the urinary bladder is the fifth most common malignancy in the United States, with an estimated 76,960 new cases and 163,900 deaths in 2016. Radical cystectomy with lymph node dissection remains the standard treatment for patients with muscle-invasive urothelial carcinoma of the bladder, and also for nonmuscle-invasive disease, refractory to intravesical therapy. The current approaches to pelvic lymph node dissections are based on the removal of lymph nodes most commonly harboring metastatic disease, notably the external iliac, obturator, and hypogastric lymph nodes. The boundaries for a standard pelvic lymph node dissection generally include the bifurcation of the common iliac vessels superiorly and the genitofemoral nerve laterally. Extended pelvic lymph node includes the removal of lymph nodes between the bifurcation of the common iliac vessels and the level of the aortic bifurcation, sometimes including distal aortic and caval nodes up to the level of the inferior mesenteric artery, as well as presacral nodes. Extended and superextended dissection has been reported to be associated with superior survival outcome.

Keywords: bladder cancer, muscle-invasive, lymph node, cystectomy

1. Introduction

Bladder cancer is the second most common genitourinary malignancy with urothelial cell carcinomas comprising nearly 90% of primary bladder tumors. Urothelial carcinoma of the urinary bladder is the fifth most common malignancy in the United States, with an estimated 76,960 new cases and 163,900 deaths in 2016 [1]. Although up to 86% of patients present with superficial or localized tumors, 20–40% present with, or progress to develop, invasive disease that carries a significant increase in the likelihood of having occult metastases [2]. Standard treatment of muscle invasive bladder cancer and refractory to intravesical chemotherapy in patients with nonmuscle invasive bladder is still radical cystectomy with lymph node dissection. Patients with muscle invasive bladder cancer have approximately 25% lymph node involvement during the radical cystectomy [3]; if lymph node involvement is observed, 10-year mortality rate can be up to 80% due to adjuvant chemotherapy [2, 3]. Although lymph node involvement portends a relatively poor prognosis, some patients exhibit long-term survival following surgery, with or without systemic chemotherapy [4]. The current approaches to pelvic lymph node dissections are based on the removal of lymph nodes most commonly harboring metastatic disease, notably the external iliac, obturator, and hypogastric lymph nodes. Standard pelvic lymph node dissection is described removing the lymph nodes including bifurcation of the common iliac vessels superiorly and the genitofemoral nerve laterally. And the limit of inferior and medial boundaries includes the obturator nerve, bladder, and internal iliac vessels medially and the endopelvic fascia, circumflex iliac veins, and Cloquet's node inferiorly [5–8] (**Figure 1**). For the standard pathological evaluation of lymph nodes to detect the presence of tumor cell after surgery, formalin fixation with hematoxylin and eosin (H&E) staining of 5-μm thick sections of each node is done. After these evaluations, nearly 25% of the patients are found to be involved with tumor in the lymph nodes during the cystectomy [9].

In the literature, the nomenclature of lymph node dissection has been variable and is defined differently by urologists. Dangle et al. divided lymph node dissection into four groups categorized as follows:

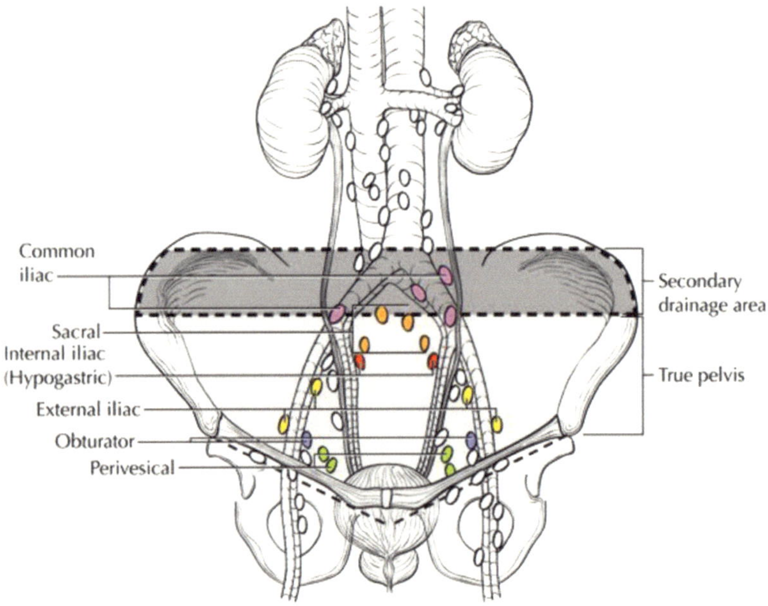

Figure 1. Regional lymph nodes of the urinary bladder. The true pelvis is the primary lymphatic drainage area for the urinary bladder. The secondary drainage area superior to the true pelvis includes the common iliac nodes and all nodes up to the level of the aortic bifurcation.

1. Limited lymphadenectomy (removal of the external iliac and obturator lymph nodes).
2. Standard lymphadenectomy (limited lymphadenectomy plus removal of the internal iliac lymph nodes).
3. Extended lymphadenectomy (standard lymphadenectomy plus removal of the common iliac and presacral lymph nodes).
4. Super-extended lymphadenectomy (extended lymphadenectomy plus removal of any additional lymph nodes above the aortic bifurcation) [10].

The boundaries of extended pelvic lymph node dissection generally include the removal of lymph nodes superior to the bifurcation of the common iliac vessels, to the level of the aortic bifurcation, sometimes including distal aortic and caval nodes up to the level of the inferior mesenteric artery and presacral nodes [11]. Extended and superextended dissection has been reported to be associated with superior survival outcome. The potential for meaningful bias, however, prohibits drawing definite conclusions [12–14].

2. Lymphatic drainage of bladder

The bladder is an extraperitoneal muscular urine reservoir that lies behind the pubic symphysis in the pelvis [15]. The lymphatic drainage of the bladder is into the obturator, external iliac, internal iliac (hypogastric), and common iliac lymph nodes. As with any region of the body, prior surgery may alter the lymphatic outflow of the region [16]. According to description of Leadbetter and Cooper in 1950, the lymphatic drainage of the bladder can be divided into six groups anatomically:

1. The visceral lymphatic plexus is located into the bladder wall, initiating inside the submucosa and extending into the muscular layer of bladder.
2. The intercalated lymph nodes that are located in the juxtavesical lymph nodes within the perivesical fat align into anterior, lateral, and posterior groups.
3. The pelvic collecting lymph nodes that drains medial side of the external iliac and hypogastric lymph nodes.
4. Regional pelvic lymph nodes that drains the external iliac, hypogastric, and presacral lymph node groups.
5. Lymphatic vessels that drains the regional pelvic lymph nodes.
6. Common iliac lymph nodes around the common iliac vessels [17].

The primary drainage of the bladder initiate from the external and internal iliac and obturator lymph nodes, secondary drainage continues from the common iliac lymph nodes, and tertiary drainage to the presacral nodes is from the trigone and posterior wall of the bladder [18]. Remarkably, a researcher from Mansoura supported the importance of the endopelvic that includes obturator and internal iliac lymph nodes as sentinels for lymphatic drainage of the bladder [19] (**Figure 1**).

3. The frequency of lymph node involvement in muscle invasive bladder cancer

Radical cystectomy with pelvic lymph node dissection remains the standard of care for patients with muscle-invasive urothelial cancer of the bladder and select patients with high-risk in nonmuscle-invasive bladder cancer. Approximately, 25% of patients with muscle-invasive bladder cancer have lymph node metastases at radical cystectomy, with 45% of patients with T3 or T4 disease, harboring nodal disease [19]. Steven and Poulsen [20] showed that 34% of their patients with lymph node-positive disease were positive in lymph nodes that are not usually included in standard lymphadenectomy. A study of autopsy including 1933 patients showed that the incidence of pelvic and retroperitoneal lymph node metastasis is 25% in 98 patients with bladder cancer [21]. Contemporary series supported that lymph node metastasis is observed in 18–24% of patients with bladder cancer [22, 23].

4. The importance of the number of positive lymph nodes

Lymph node positivity is a critical factor for disease-specific survival and a primary determinant of therapeutic course following surgery. Multi-institutional series of patients treated with radical cystectomy have shown that approximately 80% of patients with pathologic node positive disease experience disease recurrence, compared with 30% of patients with extravesical disease and pathologically negative lymph node [24–26]. Patients with regional lymph node metastasis at the time of cystectomy are at considerable risk for disease relapse and cumulative probability of survival for these patients' remains at 5–30% [27]. There is an increasing perception that extensive pelvic lymph node dissection is an important therapeutic measure associated with improvement in cancer-specific survival in both lymph node-negative and lymph node-positive patients [19, 28]. Honma et al. reported that patients with less than four positive nodes had a statistically significant survival advantage compared with four or more positive nodes, and the number of nodes removed has a significant impact on disease-specific survival in node-positive patients. The removal of 13 or more nodes had a survival benefit even in the node-positive patients [29]. If pelvic nodal involvement is proven, it should be considered a manifestation of a systemic disease. However, the independent value of pelvic lymph node dissection for survival in patients with bladder cancer remains controversial, although it has been demonstrated that pelvic lymph node dissection cures some node-positive patients [30].

Lymph node mapping studies show a significant percentage of metastases in lymph node-positive patients occurring above the common iliac bifurcation [11, 18]. Lymph node-positive patients with standard lymphadenectomy had significantly worse 5-year disease-free survival compared with lymph node-positive patients who underwent extended lymphadenectomy, and extended lymphadenectomy was an independent prognostic factor for disease-free survival [31]. Tarin et al. reported that number of positive lymph nodes was significantly associated with cancer-specific survival, whereas location of the positive node and lymph node density were not. A total of 25% of patients with pN3 disease were recurrence-free at 5 year, which is not significantly different from patients with pN1 or pN2 disease [32]. Prior to the practice of pelvic lymph node dissection, series reported dismal 5-year survival rates of 4–7% in lymph node-positive patients [33–35]. Skinner reported a 36% improvement of 5-year survival in bladder cancer patients with limited nodal disease undergoing bilateral pelvic lymph node dissection at the time of cystectomy. Skinner concluded that a "meticulous" pelvic lymph node dissection could provide cure and control of pelvic disease in some patients with regional lymph node metastases without increasing the morbidity [36]. Knowledge of lymph node status is important because it influences patient counseling and, more importantly, clinical decision-making regarding follow-up scheduling and adjuvant chemotherapy [37].

The study of International Bladder Cancer Nomogram Consortium analyzed 9064 patients who underwent radical cystectomy and lymphadenectomy for bladder cancer and reported that 1550 patients treated with surgery alone have lymph node-positive disease. As the result of this study, the authors have developed an international bladder cancer nomogram. The aim of the nomogram is using information on patient age, sex, and time from diagnosis to surgery, pathologic tumor stage and grade, tumor histological subtype, and regional lymph node status to predict recurrence risk in patients with bladder cancer after surgery. Following this study, a lot of nomogram series were published that include either total number of lymph nodes removed, number of positive lymph nodes, or lymph node density, and finally, node parameters placed in the final nomogram model [38].

Although lymph node metastasis is related to a relatively poor prognosis, some patients prove long-term survival after surgery, with or without systemic chemotherapy. Because of the different prognostic factors, stratification of lymph node-positive patients is needed to obtain more individualized risk estimations. Although some studies have reported several prognostic factors for lymph node-positive patients, predictive factors for survival in lymph node-positive patients have not been controversial [39].

5. The importance of the size of lymph nodes (extra capsular invasion of tumor, tumor burden, and lymphovascular invasion)

The extent of nodal involvement, or tumor burden, has also been reported as an independent prognostic factor for survival in patients with bladder cancer [40]. Several recent studies have also shown the prognostic influence of the degree of lymph node positivity on survival rates [25, 41, 42]. The presence of tumor cells in the endothelium-lined space is defined as lymphovascular invasion. The prognostic value of lymphovascular invasion is controversial in bladder cancer [43, 44]. Some studies reported that lymphovascular invasion was present in 36% of all the specimens in patients presenting with higher chances of metastatic disease [3, 45]. Quek et al. found a statistical correlation between lymphovascular invasion and positive surgical margins, high pathological stages, older patients, and female gender. Ten-year survival was lower in patients with lymphovascular invasion than patients without lymphovascular invasion (43 vs. 18%) [3]. Similarly, Lotan concluded in his study that lymphovascular invasion was an independent predictor of recurrence and decreased disease-specific and overall survival in lymph node-negative patients. Blood vessel invasion of tumor cells of 22 patients who had a 5-year survival of 29% [44]. In another study, 5-year survival is estimated in 56% of the 347 patients without lymphovascular invasion (p = 0.0011). Significantly higher 5-year survival was demonstrated for the 259 patients without lymphatic invasion compared to 110 with lymphatic invasion (61 vs. 39%, $p < 0.0000$). Prognosis was significantly worse in patients with perineural invasion compared with without perineural invasion (44 vs. 56%, $p = 0.0007$) [46].

6. The importance of number of removed lymph nodes

It is common knowledge that removing more nodes can improve survival. In an effort to reduce understaging and maximize survival, many studies have tried to establish a minimum number of lymph nodes needed to be taken at the time of radical cystectomy [40, 47, 48]. Several studies have indicated that the number of lymph nodes removed is a prognostic factor in bladder cancer patients [7, 46, 47]. Researchers have tried to identify the minimum necessary number of lymph nodes needed to be removed at radical cystectomy. However, the analysis of a large tertiary care center's database revealed that the probability of survival continues to rise as the number of lymph nodes removed increases and that no minimum number of lymph nodes can be determined [48]. Although several groups defined a minimum number of lymph nodes to be removed to confer a survival benefit [40, 49], Koppie et al. reported that the probability of survival rises as the number of lymph node removed increases [48]. Herr reported in his study that lymph node-negative patients have increased survival and correlated with the number of nodes removed, regardless of the stage of the tumor. As a result of this study, the authors advised a minimum of nine lymph nodes should be removed [42]. Stein et al. [41] demonstrated that patients with 15 or more nodes removed had better recurrence-free survival than did those with less than 15 nodes removed. Leissner reported in his study that adjuvant chemotherapy has positive effects on survival for lymph node-positive patients or with extravesical disease, if 16 nodes were removed. Moreover, when lymph node positivity is observed, survival increases, if the number of lymph node-positive was ≤5 [44]. Konety et al. [47] reported decreased risk of mortality when 10–14 lymph nodes were removed. The Southwest Oncology Group study 8710 showed that the survival advantage conferred by the removal of 10 or more nodes was found even in node-negative patients [50].

Fleischmann et al. performed only standard lymphadenectomy and removed a mean of 23 pelvic lymph nodes. But when patients were divided into quartiles by the number of nodes examined, researchers could not find any significant differences in recurrence-free and overall survival rates [51].

7. Factors that affect the number of removed lymph nodes in cystectomy

Different factors affect the actual number of lymph nodes removed and/or examined. A lot of studies about the number of lymphadenectomy is high, but all have the limitations of retrospective studies, and the boundaries of lymphadenectomy were variable and the mean numbers of removed nodes were different. Because of the different surgeons and pathologists, the number of removed lymph nodes and evaluated number of lymph node and detected positive number of lymph nodes may vary [52]. In the surgical series, the number of retrieved lymph nodes can be influenced by many factors, including the extent of pelvic lymph node dissection, intraoperative decisions regarding the amount of tissue to remove within each region of the pelvic lymph node, surgeon's experience, and presentation of pathologic specimens [53].

8. What should be the limit in pelvic lymph node dissection?

There still exists no consensus about the optimal boundaries of lymph node dissection, the number of removed lymph nodes, and procedure's prognostic and therapeutic role for patients who underwent radical cystectomy for muscle-invasive bladder cancer, although the importance of lymph node status is proven for treatment of the bladder cancer [18, 49]. The histopathological results and the extent of lymph node removal have significance as prognostic criteria and thus as indicators for adjuvant therapy [8, 19, 28].

Nowadays, the European Association of Urology and the American Urological Association guidelines could not advise clear recommendations about the boundaries of lymphadenectomy and the number of removed lymph nodes [54]. The International Consultation on Urological Diseases 2012 guidelines recommend the removal of all lymphatic tissue around the common iliac, external iliac, internal iliac, and obturator group bilaterally because one-third of all positive nodes are located around the common iliac artery [55].

Poulsen et al. [6] observed that extending the pelvic lymph node dissection to the bifurcation of the aorta improved survival in patients with organ-confined (pT3a or less) disease.

Bi et al. reported a meta-analysis of six studies. They compared patients who underwent extended lymph node dissection with nonextended lamp node dissection. They reported that extended lymph node dissection have better recurrent-free survival than patients who underwent nonextended lymph node dissection. And also, in a subgroup analysis, they showed that patient who underwent extended lymph node dissection have better recurrent-free survival than nonextended patients in both patients with lymph node positive and negative [56].

Crozier reported that nonurothelial cancers are more advanced tumors than urothelial cancers at the time of diagnosis. According to their results, more aggressive surgical treatment must be performed for patients with nonurothelial muscle invasive cancer. Because of the potential survival benefits for these patients, they recommend standard extended lymphadenectomy in patients diagnosed with nonurothelial muscle invasive cancer [57].

At present, the limitation of exact boundaries of pelvic lymph node dissection remains controversial both in the literature and in the guidelines [58]. It is obvious that a pelvic lymph node dissection must be performed during cystectomy; however, in some studies, pelvic lymph node dissection was not performed in 8, 11, and 60% of patients [59–61]. On the other hand, in another recent SEER analysis performed between 1992 and 2003, 3603 cystectomies were analyzed. In this study, including the hospitals, cystectomies were divided into groups according to the number of lymph nodes removed. The authors demonstrated that only 0–4 nodes were removed in 88.9% of patients in low-node count hospitals and 52.8% of cases in the high-node count hospitals; likewise, 10–14 nodes were removed in 7.2% in low-node count hospitals and 14.2% of patients in the medium- and high-node count hospitals [61].

9. Morbidity and mortality of pelvic lymph node dissection

Cystectomy is a one of major surgical procedure among urological operations with potential complications often related to the urinary diversion. However, a pelvic lymph node dissection does not have any effect on overall morbidity; it can increase operation time and sometimes facilitate the execution of the cystectomy. The different parameters may affect the morbidity related to pelvic lymph node dissection. Especially, in experienced hands, removing of pelvic lymph node did not increase operative morbidity and using the anatomical approach may decrease perioperative complications and perioperative mortality [62]. Moreover, increasing the number of nodes removed did not increase morbidity. Some complications related to lymphadenectomy, such as lymphoceles and lymphoedemas, were reported in 2% of patients with <16 lymph nodes removed and 1% with 16 nodes removed [63]. As a result, pelvic lymph node dissection is recommended if patients have no absolute contraindication and fit enough to undergo a radical cystectomy, regardless of age and comorbidities.

10. Conclusion

Presence of lymph node metastasis is associated with poor recurrence-free and overall survival. Cystectomy with pelvic lymph node dissection is crucial for appropriate staging, removal of micrometastatic disease, and identifying candidates for adjuvant chemotherapy in patients with muscle invasive bladder cancer. Although there is still no consensus about the limit of pelvic lymph node dissection, extended lymphadenectomy must performed in patients with high risk of metastasis because of the potential survival benefit of the lymphadenectomy.

Author details

Mustafa Ozan Horsanali* and Kutan Ozer

*Address all correspondence to: drozanhorsanali@yahoo.com

Urology Department, Izmir Katip Celebi University Ataturk Training and Research Hospital, Izmir, Turkey

References

[1] National Cancer Institute, Surveillance, Epidemiology, and End Results Program. SEER Stat Fact Sheets: Number of new cases and death in 2016. Available from: http://seer.cancer.gov/statfacts/html/all.html.

[2] Stein JP, Lieskovsky G, Cote R, Groshen S, Feng AC, et al. Radical cystectomy in the treatment of invasive bladder cancer: long-term results in 1,054 patients. J Clin Oncol 2001;19:666–75.

[3] Quek ML, Sanderson KM, Daneshmand S, Stein JP. The importance of an extended lymphadenectomy in the management of high-grade invasive bladder cancer. Expert Rev Anticancer Ther 2004;4:1007–16.

[4] Millikan R, Dinney C, Swanson D, Sweeney P, Ro JY, et al. Integrated therapy for locally advanced bladder cancer: final report of a randomized trial of cystectomy plus adjuvant M-VAC versus cystectomy with both preoperative and postoperative M-VAC. J Clin Oncol 2001;19:4005–13.

[5] Nieh P, Marshall F. Surgery of bladder cancer. In Wein AJ, Kavoussi LR, Novick AC, Partin AW, Peters CA, eds, Campbell- Walsh Urology, Philadelphia: Saunders Elsevier, 2007: 2479–505.

[6] Poulsen A, Horn T, Steven K. Radical cystectomy: extending limits of pelvic lymph node dissection improves survival for patients with bladder cancer confined to the bladder wall. J Urol 1998;160:2015–9.

[7] Dhar NB, Klein EA, Reuther AM, Thalmann GN, Madersbacher S, et al. Outcome after radical cystectomy with limited or extended pelvic lymph node dissection. J Urol 2008;179:873–8.

[8] Sharir S, Fleshner N. Lymph node assessment and lymphadenectomy in bladder cancer. J Surg Onc 2009;99:225–31.

[9] Stein JP, Skinner D. The role of lymphadenectomy in high-grade invasive bladder cancer. Urol Clin North Am 2005;32:187–97.

[10] Dangle PP, Bahnson RR, Pohar KS. How close are we to establishing standards of lymphadenectomy for invasive bladder cancer? Ther Adv Urol 2009;1(3):167–74.

[11] Roth B, Wissmeyer MP, Zehnder P, Birkhäuser FD, Thalmann GN, et al. A new multi-modality technique accurately maps the primary lymphatic landing sites of the bladder. Eur Urol 2010;57(2):205–11.

[12] Alfred Witjes J, Lebret T, Compérat EM, Cowan NC, De Santis M, et al. Updated 2016 EAU guidelines on muscle-invasive and metastatic bladder cancer. Eur Urol 2016 Jun 30. pii: S0302-2838(16)30290-1. doi: 10.1016/j.eururo.2016.06.020. [Epub ahead of print].

[13] Morgan TM, Barocas DA, Penson DF, Chang SS, Ni S, et al. Lymph node yield at radical cystectomy predicts mortality in node-negative and not node-positive patients. Urology 2012;80:632–40.

[14] Tilki D, Brausi M, Colombo R, Evans CP, Fradet Y, et al. Lymphadenectomy for bladder cancer at the time of radical cystectomy. Eur Urol 2013;64:266–76.

[15] Fowler CJ, Griffiths D, de Groat WC. The neural control of micturition. Nat Rev Neurosci 2008 Jun;9(6):453–66.

[16] Abol-Enein H, El-Baz M, Abd El-Hameed MA, Abdel-Latif M, Ghoneim MA. Lymph node involvement in patients with bladder cancer treated with radical cystectomy: a patho-anatomical study—a single center experience. J Urol 2004;172(5):1818–21.

[17] Leadbetter WF, Cooper JF. Regional gland dissection for carcinoma of the bladder: a technique for one-stage cystectomy, gland dissection, and bilateral ureteroenterostomy. J Urol 1950;63:242–60.

[18] Vazina A, Dugi D, Shariat SF, Evans J, Link R, et al. Stage specific lymph node metastasis mapping in radical cystectomy specimens. J Urol 2004;171:1830–4.

[19] Leissner J, Ghoneim MA, Abol-Enein H, Thüroff JW, Franzaring L, et al. Extended radical lymphadenectomy in patients with urothelial bladder cancer: results of a prospective multicenter study. J Urol 2004;171:139–44.

[20] Steven K, Poulsen AL. Radical cystectomy and extended pelvic lymphadenectomy: survival of patients with lymph node metastasis above the bifurcation of the common iliac vessels treated with surgery only. J Urol 2007;178:1218–24.

[21] Colston JA, Leadbetter WF. Infiltrating carcinoma of the bladder. J Urol 1936;36:669.

[22] Hautmann RE, Gschwend JE, de Petriconi RC, Kron M, Volkmer BG. Cystectomy for transitional cell carcinoma of the bladder: results of a surgery only series in the neobladder era. J Urol 2006;176:486–92.

[23] Madersbacher S, Hochreiter W, Burkhard F, Thalmann GN, Danuser H, et al. Radical cystectomy for bladder cancer today—a homogeneous series without neoadjuvant therapy. J Clin Oncol 2003;21:686–90.

[24] Karakiewicz PI, Shariat SF, Palapattu GS, Gilad AE, Lotan Y, et al. Nomogram for predicting disease recurrence after radical cystectomy for transitional cell carcinoma of the bladder. J Urol 2006;176:1354–61, discussion 1361–2.

[25] Shariat SF, Karakiewicz PI, Palapattu GS, Amiel GE, Lotan Y, et al. Nomograms provide improved accuracy for predicting survival after radical cystectomy. Clin Cancer Res 2006;12:6663–76.

[26] Karakiewicz PI, Shariat SF, Palapattu GS, Perrotte P, Lotan Y, et al. Precystectomy nomogram for prediction of advanced bladder cancer stage. Eur Urol 2006;50:1254–62, discussion 1261–2.

[27] Palapattu GS, Shariat SF, Karakiewicz PI, Bastian PJ, Rogers CG, et al. Cancer-specific outcomes in patients with pT0 disease following radical cystectomy. J Urol 2006;175: 1645–9, Discussion 9.

[28] Buscarini M, Josephson DY, Stein JP. Lymphadenectomy in bladder cancer: a review. Urol Int 2007;79:191–9.

[29] Honma I, Masumori N, Sato E, Maeda T, Hirobe M, et al. Removal of more lymph nodes may provide better outcome, as well as more accurate pathologic findings, in patients with bladder cancer—analysis of role of pelvic lymph node dissection. Urology 2006;68 (3):543–8.

[30] Dalbagni G, Genega E, Hashibe M, Zhang ZF, Russo P, et al. Cystectomy for bladder cancer: a contemporary series. J Urol 2001;165:1111–6.

[31] Abol-Enein H, Tilki D, Mosbah A, El-Baz M, Shokeir A, et al. Does the extent of lymphadenectomy in radical cystectomy for bladder cancer influence disease-free survival? A prospective single-center study. Eur Urol 2011:60;572–7.

[32] Tarin T, Power NE, Ehdaie B, Sfakianos JP, Silberstein JL, et al. Lymph node-positive bladder cancer treated with radical cystectomy and lymphadenectomy: effect of the level of node positivity. Our Urol 2012:61;1025–30.

[33] Smith JA, Whitmore Jr WF. Regional lymph node metastasis from bladder cancer. J Urol 1981;126:591–3.

[34] Guiliani L, Giberti C, Martorana G, Bonamini A, Natta GD, et al. Results of radical cystectomy for primary bladder cancer: retrospective study of more than 200 cases. Urology 1985;26:243–8.

[35] Pagano F, Bassi P, Galetti TP, Meneghini A, Milani C, et al. Results of contemporary radical cystectomy for invasive bladder cancer: a clinicopathological study with an emphasis on the inadequacy of the tumor, nodes and metastases classification. J Urol 1991;145:45–50.

[36] Skinner DG. Management of invasive bladder cancer: a meticulous pelvic node dissection can make a difference. J Urol 1982;128:34–6.

[37] Feifer AH, Taylor JM, Tarin TV, Herr HW. Maximizing cure for muscle-invasive bladder cancer: integration of surgery and chemotherapy. Eur Urol 2011;59:978–84.

[38] Bochner BH, Kattan MW, Vora KC. Postoperative nomogram predicting risk of recurrence after radical cystectomy for bladder cancer. J Clin Oncol 2006;24:3967–72.

[39] Herr HW, Donat SM. Outcome of patients with grossly node positive bladder cancer after pelvic lymph node dissection and radical cystectomy. J Urol 2001;165:62–4.

[40] Mills RD, Turner WH, Fleischmann A, Markwalder R, Thalmann GN, et al. Pelvic lymph node metastases from bladder cancer: outcome in 83 patients after radical cystectomy and pelvic lymphadenectomy. J Urol 2001;166:19–23.

[41] Stein J, Cai J, Groshen S, Skinner DG. Risk factors for patients with pelvic lymph node metastases following radical cystectomy with en bloc pelvic lymphadenectomy: concept of lymph node density. J Urol 2003;170:35–41.

[42] Herr HW, Bochner BH, Dalbagni G, Donat SM, Reuter VE, et al. Impact of the number of lymph nodes retrieved on outcome in patients with muscle invasive bladder cancer. J Urol 2002;167:1295–8.

[43] Cheng L, Neumann RM, Scherer BG, Weaver AL, Leibovich BC, et al. Tumor size predicts the survival of patients with pathologic stage T2 bladder carcinoma: a critical evaluation of the depth of muscle invasion. Cancer 1999;15(85):2638–47.

[44] Leissner J, Koeppen C, Wolf HK. Prognostic significance of vascular and perineural invasion in urothelial bladder cancer treated with radical cystectomy. J Urol 2003;169: 955–60.

[45] Lotan Y, Gupta A, Shariat SF, Palapattu GS, Vazina A, et al. Lymphovascular invasion is independently associated with overall survival, cause-specific survival, and local and distant recurrence in patients with negative lymph nodes at radical cystectomy. J Clin Oncol 2005;23:6533–9.

[46] Bassi P, Ferrante GD, Piazza N, Spinadin R, Carando R, et al. Prognostic factors of outcome after radical cystectomy for bladder cancer: a retrospective study of a homogeneous patient cohort. J Urol 1999;161:1494–7.

[47] Konety BR, Joslyn SA, O'Donnell MA. Extent of pelvic lymphadenectomy and its impact on outcome in patients diagnosed with bladder cancer: analysis of data from the Surveillance, Epidemiology and End Results Program data base. J Urol 2003;169:946–50.

[48] Koppie TM, Vickers AJ, Vora K, Dalbagni G, Bochner BH. Standardization of pelvic lymphadenectomy performed at radical cystectomy: can we establish a minimum number of lymph nodes that should be removed?. Cancer 2006;107:2368–74.

[49] Capitanio U, Suardi N, Shariat SF, Lotan Y, Palapattu GS, et al. Assessing the minimum number of lymph nodes needed at radical cystectomy in patients with bladder cancer. BJU Int 2009;103:1359–62.

[50] Herr HW, Faulkner JR, Grossman B, Natale RB, deVere White R, et al. Surgical factors influence bladder cancer outcomes: a cooperative group report. J Clin Oncol 2004;22: 2781–9.

[51] Fleischmann A, Thalmann GN, Markwalder R, Studer UE. Extracapsular extension of pelvic lymph node metastases from urothelial carcinoma of the bladder is an independent prognostic factor. J Clin Oncol 2005;23:2358–65.

[52] Herr HW. Extent of surgery and pathology evaluation has an impact on bladder cancer outcomes after radical cystectomy. Urology 2003;61:105–8.

[53] Heidenreich A, Pfister D. Anatomic extent of pelvic lymphadenectomy in bladder cancer. Eur Urol Suppl 2010;9:419–23.

[54] Stenzl A, Cowan NC, De Santis M, Kuczyk MA, Merseburger AS, et al. Treatment of muscle invasive and metastatic bladder cancer: update of the EAU guidelines. Eur Urol 2011;59:1009–18.

[55] Gakis G, Efstathiou J, Lerner SP, Cookson MS, Keegan KA, et al. ICUD-EAU International Consultation on Bladder Cancer 2012: radical cystectomy and bladder preservation for muscle-invasive urothelial carcinoma of the bladder. Eur Urol 2013;63:45–57.

[56] Bi L, Huang H, Fan X, Li K, Xu K, et al. Extended vs non-extended pelvic lymph node dissection and their influence on recurrence-free survival in patients undergoing radical cystectomy for bladder cancer: a systematic review and meta-analysis of comparative studies. BJU Int 2014;113:39–48.

[57] Crozier J, Demkiw S, Lawrentschuk N. Utility of lymphadenectomy following cystectomy for non-urothelial bladder cancer. Minerva Urol Nefrol 2016;68:185–91.

[58] Stenzl A, Cowan NC, De Santis M, Jakse G, Kuczyk MA, et al. The updated EAU guidelines on muscle invasive and metastatic bladder cancer. Eur Urol 2009;55(4):815–25.

[59] Herr H, Lee C, Chang S, Lerner S. Bladder Cancer Collaborative Group. Standardization of radical cystectomy and pelvic lymph node dissection for bladder cancer: a collaborative group report. J Urol 2004;171:1823–8.

[60] Knap MM, Lundbeck F, Overgaard J. The role of pelvic lymph node dissection as a predictive and prognostic factor in bladder cancer. Eur J Cancer 2003;39(5):604–13.

[61] Hollenbeck BK, Ye Z, Wong SL, Montie JE, Birkmeyer JD. Hospital lymph node counts and survival after radical cystectomy. Cancer 2008;15(112):806–12.

[62] Lerner SP, Skinner DG, Lieskovsky G, Boyd SD, Groshen SL, et al. The rationale for en bloc pelvic lymph node dissection for bladder cancer patients with nodal metastases: long-term results. J Urol 1993;149:758–64.

[63] Leissner J, Hohenfellner R, Thuroff JW, Wolf HK. Lymphadenectomy in patients with transitional cell carcinoma of the urinary bladder: significance for staging and prognosis. BJU Int 2000;85:817–23.

Chapter 6

Genital Organs-Sparing Radical Cystectomy in Female Patients with Muscle Invasive Urothelial Carcinoma of the Bladder

Hosni Khairy Salem

Additional information is available at the end of the chapter

http://dx.doi.org/10.5772/67759

Abstract

There has been considerable interest in urethral-sparing cystectomy and preservation of the gynecological tract to maintain continence mechanism, sexual function, and reproductive function in young patients who undergo radical cystectomy for muscle-invasive bladder cancer and this new technique gained acceptance in many centers. The issue of oncological safety of a urethra and anterior vaginal wall-sparing cystectomy in selected patients has been addressed by several authors. The chapter will discuss the following items: (I) Technique of genital-sparing radical cystectomy in female patients with muscle invasive transitional cell carcinoma of the bladder. (II) Definition and rationale of genital-sparing radical cystectomy in female patients. (III) Rational and value of urethral preservation in genital-sparing cystectomy in female patients with urothelial carcinoma. (IV) Previous reports about genital-sparing cystectomy in patients with urothelial carcinoma. (V) Value of preservation of the internal genital organs in female patients undergoing radical cystectomy.

Keywords: genital-sparing, radical cystectomy, female, transitional cell carcinoma, urinary diversion

1. Introduction

Radical cystectomy in females includes an anterior exenteration, i.e., removal of the bladder, urethra, uterus, fallopian tubes, ovaries, and anterior wall of the vagina. The oncological necessity for removal of the internal genital organs has been questioned [1].

There has been considerable interest in urethral-sparing cystectomy and preservation of the gynecological tract to maintain continence mechanism, sexual function, and reproductive function in young patients who undergo radical cystectomy for muscle-invasive bladder cancer and gained acceptance in many centers [2–5].

The issue of oncological safety of a urethra and anterior vaginal wall-sparing cystectomy in selected patients has been addressed by several authors [2–7].

The scientific rationale of internal genital organ preservation during radical cystectomy in women was based on studies documented the low incidence of internal genitalia involvement in female bladder cancer [4–7].

With increasing survival from bladder cancer, quality of life (QOL) and quality of sexuality considered now an important end point after such type of surgery particularly in young female patients diagnosed with bladder cancer and eager to preserve fertility [4, 5].

Studies concerning genital-sparing cystectomy are few and their limitations included; few cases [4–6], retrospective [8, 9], limited long-term follow-up [4, 5, 7], incomplete functional and oncological outcome [6, 7], and finally included cases with nonorthotopic diversion [5–7, 10].

2. Technique of genital-sparing radical cystectomy in female patients with muscle invasive transitional cell carcinoma of the bladder

2.1. Preoperative assessment

History taking included; voiding and sexual function questionnaire while staging of the tumor included; clinical examination for clinical staging of the tumor and investigation like pelvic-abdominal ultrasound and CT scanning.

A thorough gynecological checkup includes a vaginal pap smear and transvaginal ultrasound. Cystoscopy was done (with biopsy from the tumor itself, bladder neck, trigone, and posterior wall) to exclude carcinoma *in situ* (CIS). Sexual function was assessed through specific questions about sexual desire (libido), orgasmic problems, and dyspareunia. Continence was assessed through voiding diary and reporting day and night continence and voiding frequency.

2.2. Preoperative preparation

Bowel preparation is started one day before the operation and consisted of two colonic return flow-enemas. All patients received prophylactic antibiotics (cephalosporin and metronidazole) 1 hour before operation and SC heparin the morning of the operation with medical leg stocking immediately preoperative.

2.3. Position and anethesia and incision

Bilateral leg compression stocking are applied.

The patient is placed in dorsal Trendelenburg position with overextension of the pelvis to open the area between the umbilicus and the pelvis.

The preferred types of anesthesia are either general anesthesia or combined general and epidural anesthesia. A 20 French Foley catheter is introduced in the urethra and the balloon inflated to 20 cc. Sponge is introduced in the vagina. A lower midline subumbilical incision is made.

2.4. Lymphadenectomy

Bilateral pelvic lymphadenectomy is performed from the site of crossing of the ureter over the common iliac artery (proximally) to the lateral circumflex iliac vein, inguinal ligament, and node of Cloquet (distally) and from the genitofemoral nerve crossing the psoas muscle (laterally) to the bladder (medially) and including the hypogastric, presciatic, presacral, and obturator fossa nodes. If we found grossly palpable and suspicious node, we extend the margins of lymphadenectomy till paraaortic lymph nodes and consider abandoning the genital-sparing technique to standard.

2.5. Posterior dissection

Transverse or U-shaped incision is made in the peritoneum of the Cul-de-sac between the bladder and the uterus (**Figure 1**).

Dissecting the fatty and fibrovascular tissue between the uterus and the bladder as far inferiorly as the level of the cervix will be the next step (**Figure 2**).

The ureter is dissected from the iliac bifurcation proximally to the posterior bladder wall distally (juxtavesical ureter) where it is crossed by the uterine artery, which is preserved.

The ureters are clipped and transected, cut margins are sent for frozen section examination (**Figure 3**).

Lateral vesical pedicles are secured and divided. While dissecting lateral to the bladder, it is advisable to avoid injury to paravaginal tissues so that the branches of the pelvic nerve plexus

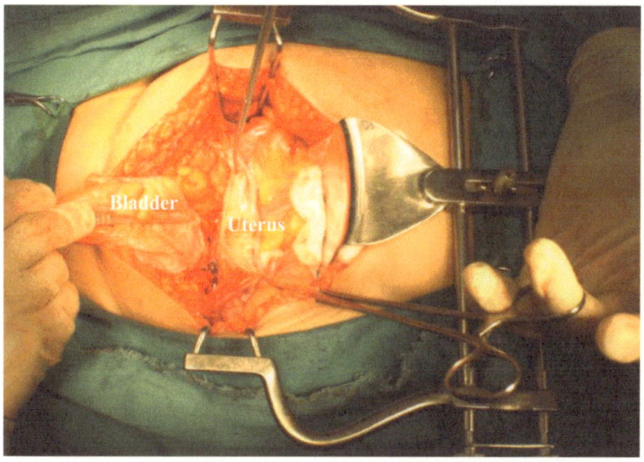

Figure 1. Urachus is divided, transverse or U-shaped incision is made in the peritoneum of the Cul-de-Sac between the bladder and the uterus.

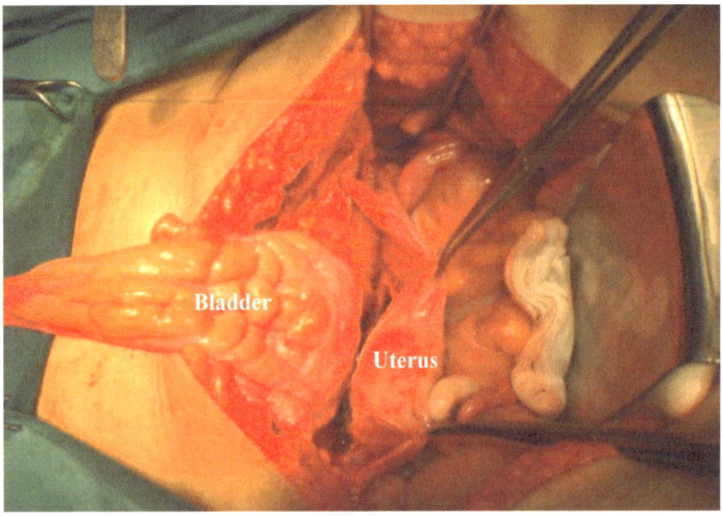

Figure 2. Dissecting the fatty and fibrovascular tissue between the uterus and the bladder as far inferiorly as possible (level of the cervix).

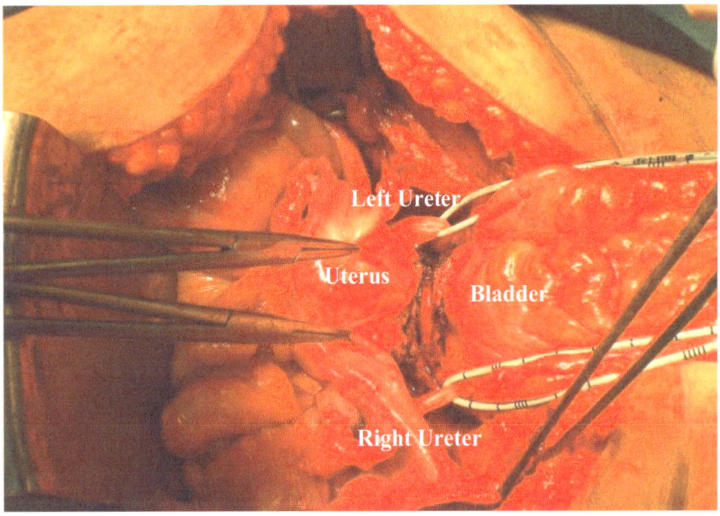

Figure 3. The ureter is dissected from the iliac bifurcation proximally to the posterior bladder wall distally (juxtavesical ureter), clipped and transected, cut margins are sent for frozen section examination.

(which course laterally to the vagina) can be preserved. Cardinal ligaments (connecting lateral surface of the cervix and the vagina to the pelvic wall) left intact.

2.6. Anterior dissection

Endopelvic fascia is incised close to the bladder neck, then we identify the vesico-urethral junction (bladder neck) by slight traction on the balloon,and putting two small sponge sticks (peanuts) on either side of the balloon (**Figure 4**).

http://dx.doi.org/10.5772/67759

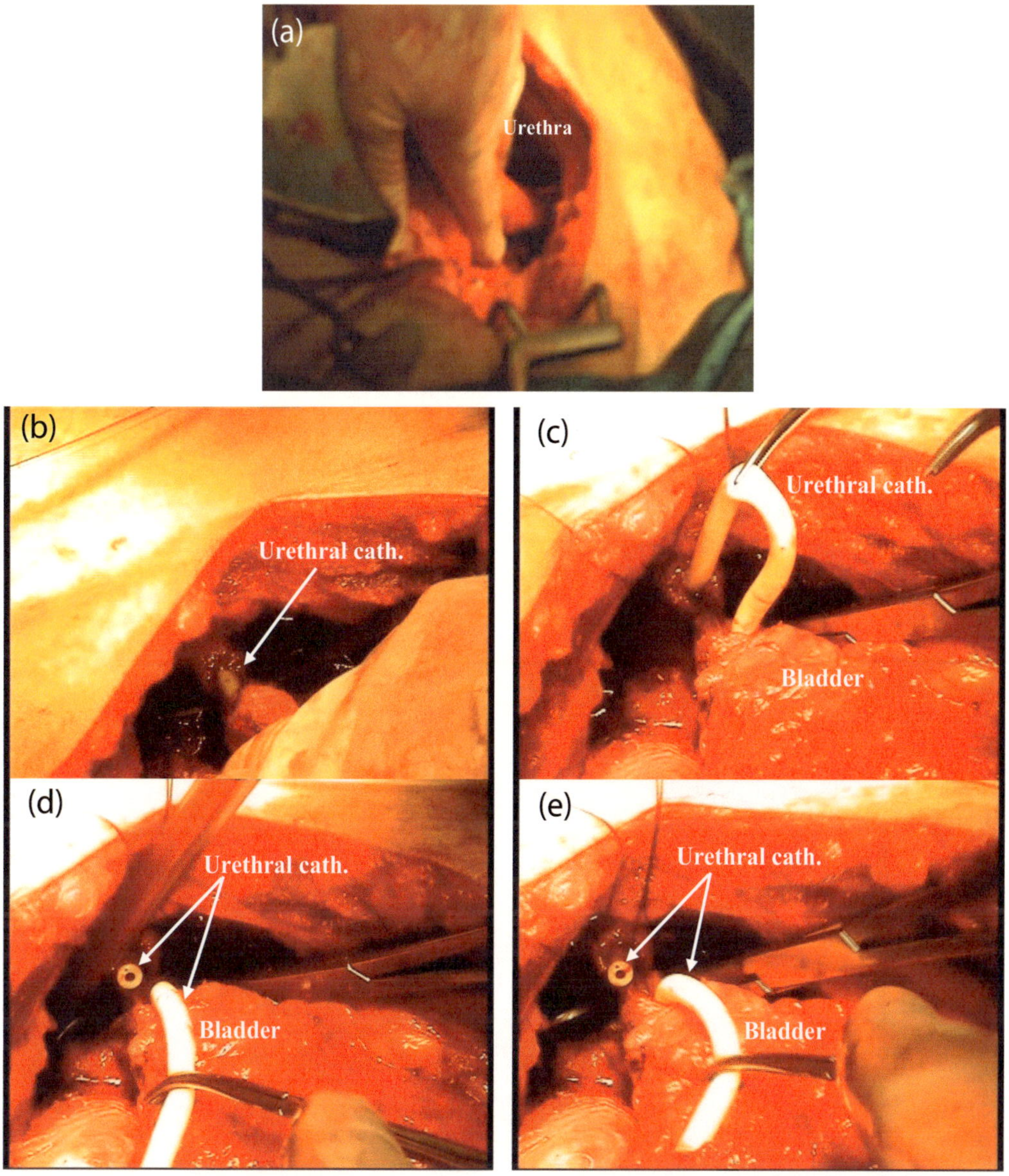

Figure 4. Endopelvic fascia incised close to the bladder neck, identify the vesicourethral junction (bladder neck). The dorsal venous complex is ligated and divided, the urethra is dissected from its attachments to the vagina and is hooked with a right angle clamp. The anterior wall of the urethra is divided sharply, the catheter pulled out, clamped proximally to prevent balloon deflation, and divided and then the posterior wall is divided. Urethral cut margins are sent for frozen section examinations.

The dorsal venous complex is ligated and divided. Ligation of the dorsal vein complex in female patients differs from male patients where other options are available to manage.

By sharp dissection, the urethra is dissected from its attachments to the vagina 0.5 cm below the bladder neck and is hooked with a right angle clamp.

The anterior wall of the urethra is divided sharply 0.5 cm below the bladder neck, the catheter pulled out, clamped proximally to prevent balloon deflation, and divided and then the posterior wall is divided with care to avoid injury of the vaginal wall.

Urethral cut margins are sent for frozen section examinations.

Care is taken not to dissect anterior and distal to the level of the transection, to ensure preservation of the pubourethral and urethropelvic ligaments, and to decrease the possibility of vaginal wall descent and pelvic prolapse.

2.7. Developing vesicovaginal and vesicourethral space

This is the most difficult and bloody part of the operation.

By gentle traction on the catheter, the bladder neck is dissected off the vaginal vault, sharp and blunt dissection continued upwards between the bladder and the vagina to connect with the previously developed posterior plane carefully without injuring the vault of the vagina and paravaginal tissues (**Figure 5**).

Six sutures of 3-0 vicryl are placed in the distal cut end of the urethra and retained for later anastomosis to the neobladder (**Figure 6**).

Alternatively, the vesicovaginal space can be developed in antegrade manner starting from above at the level of the junction between the cervix and the anterior vagina (whitish plane) (**Figure 7**).

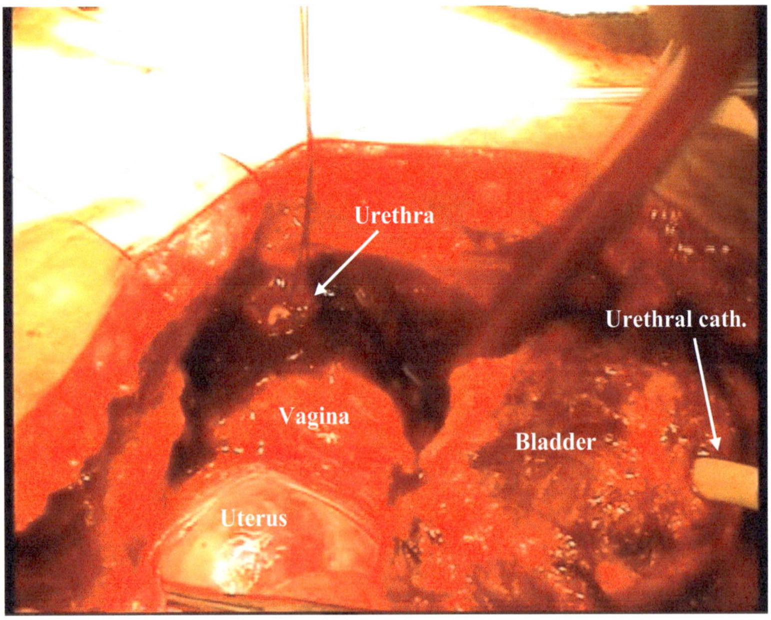

Figure 5. By gentle traction on the catheter, the bladder neck is dissected off the vaginal vault, sharp and blunt dissection continued upwards between the bladder and the vagina to connect with the previously developed posterior plane carefully.

http://dx.doi.org/10.5772/67759

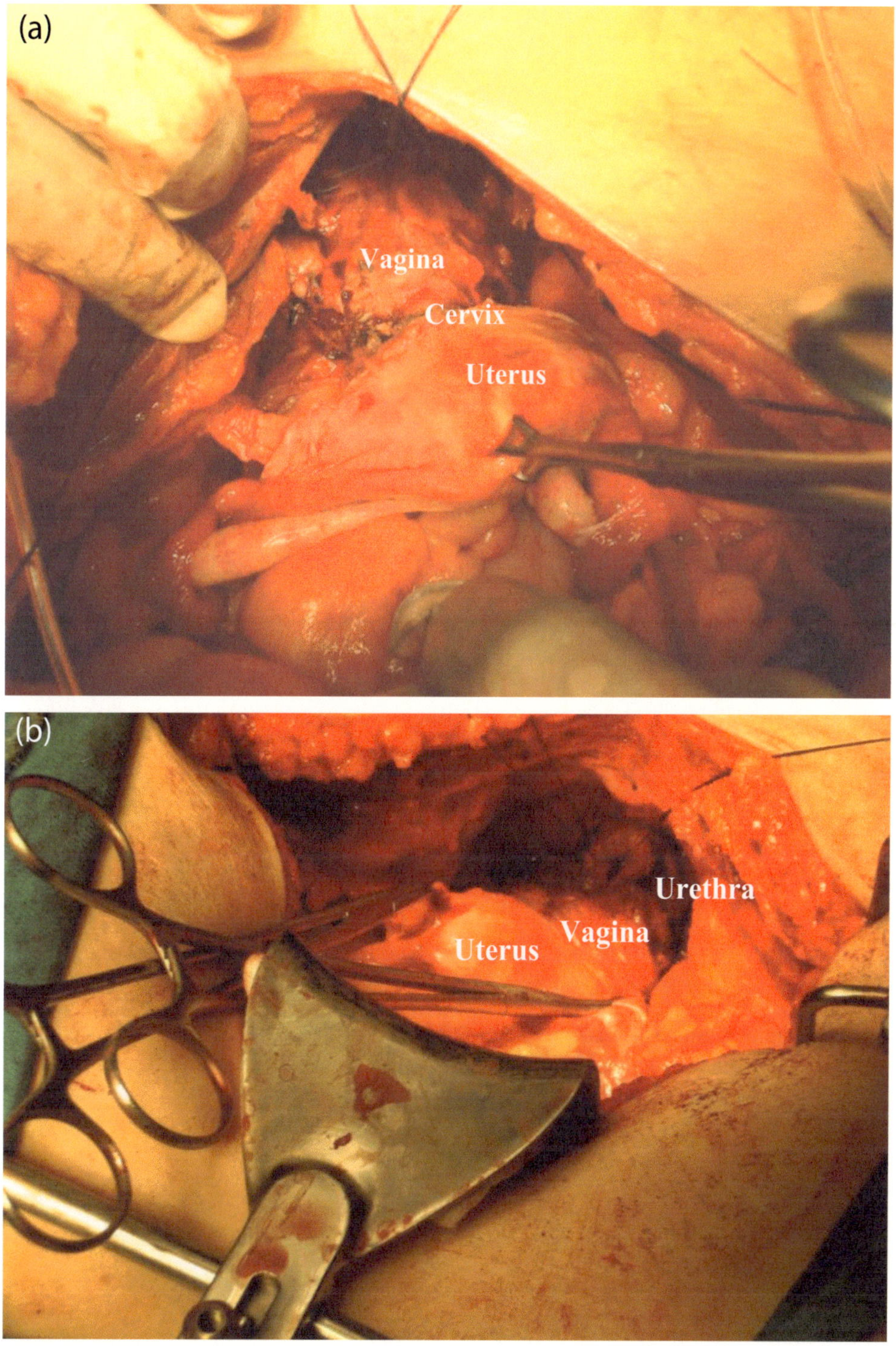

Figure 6. (a) Final picture after removal of the bladder and (b) six sutures of 3-0 vicryl are placed in the distal cut end of the urethra and retained for later anastomosis to the neobladder.

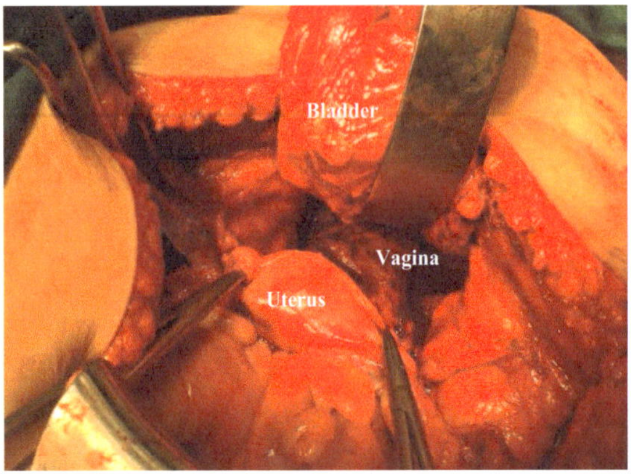

Figure 7. Alternatively, the vesicovaginal space can be developed in antegrade manner starting from above at the level of the junction between the cervix and the anterior vagina (whitish plane).

Dissection close to the vaginal wall will avoid injury to the neurovascular bundles supplying vagina, urethra, and clitoris.

2.8. Urinary diversion

A segment of 60 cm of the ileum is isolated on a vascular pedicle from a point 15–20 cm proximal to the ileocaecal junction. The bowel is detubularized and reconfigured in a W pouch.

The ureters are implanted creating serosa-lined tunnels.

The neobladder is anastomosed to the urethra using the preplaced vicryl sutures over a 20-French Foley catheter (**Figure 8**). The anastomotic site must sit broadly on the pelvic floor and should be away from the most dependent part of the reservoir. In one patient, an ileocaecal neobladder was created.

It is not essential to use a well-vascularized omental flap behind the reconstructed pouch in our cases because the preserved vagina was not opened (no suture lines).

The initial capacity was assessed by filling the bladder through the Foley catheter, and the initial capacity was approximately 120 cc after filling.

Two ureteral stents were left.

Drains are placed and the incision is closed in layers.

2.9. Postoperative care and follow up

Ureteral stent is removed 7–9 days postoperatively before discharge.

Urethral catheter is removed 2 weeks postoperatively if the pouchogram showed no extravasations.

Pouch wash with sodium bicarbonate starting from the 4th day postoperatively. Patient is advised to void by pelvic floor relaxation in sitting position at 3-hour interval day and night,

http://dx.doi.org/10.5772/67759

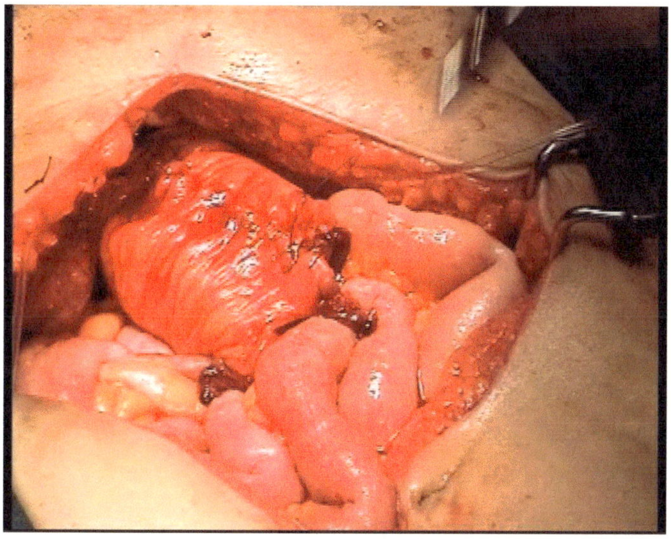

Figure 8. The final picture after fishing closure of the orthotopic pouch with poucho-urethral anastomosis.

increase the voiding intervals gradually with time (retain urine for 3–4 hours) to obtain bladder capacity of 500 cc.

Patient sexual function, voiding patterns, and continence are assessed by means of a validated questionnaire and personal interviews. Sexual function was assessed through specific questions about sexual desire (libido), orgasmic problems, and dyspareunia. Continence was assessed through voiding diary and reporting day and night continence and voiding frequency.

The patient is considered to be continent if she required not more than one pad during the night or the day. Postvoid residual urine is assessed by means of ultrasound or self-catheterization after spontaneous voiding.

Pathological examination of the specimen is done to assess the stage, grade, and lymph node status.

Follow up at 3-month interval should include: personal interviews (sexual function with three questions related to dyspareunia, vaginal lubrication and overall satisfaction), voiding patterns, continence (number of pads used), chemistry, gynecological examination, test for residual urine, and CT examination.

3. Definition and rationale of genital-sparing radical cystectomy in female patients

In the past, radical cystectomy in females included an anterior exenteration, i.e., removal of the bladder, urethra, uterus, fallopian tubes, ovaries, and anterior wall of the vagina. The reasons for removing the adnexa (in radical cystectomy in female patients) are not clear and have been questioned because bladder cancer rarely extends to these organs. The risk of internal genitalia involvement in female cystectomy specimen was reported to be low whether primary or secondary. Uterine involvement in patients with urothelial cancer has been reported in 1/37 and in 2/40 radical cystectomy specimens in Groutz et al. and Chang et al. studies, respectively [11, 12].

In another study included more than 600, the rate of concomitant gynecological organ involvement has been reported to be 2.6% [13].

In our previous studies, we examined cystectomy specimens from 360 consecutive female patients with bladder cancer, pathologically for internal genitalia involvement. Uterine involvement was observed in one case of TCC (pT4, grade III). Uterine benign pathology was detected in 25 cases. All patients had normal ovaries regardless of tumor site or stage while the vagina was involved in 11 cases. Ten percent of the patients had urethral involvement (all had TCC). During late follow up of 50 patients (included two cases with uterine preservation, and in all cases, at least one ovary was preserved), no single ovarian or uterine recurrence was reported [14, 15].

4. Rational and value of urethral preservation in genital-sparing cystectomy in female patients with urothelial carcinoma

Urethral preservation under specific criteria of tumor site and extension is quite safe and facilitates orthotopic reconstruction with spontaneous voiding and improves the quality of life in such patients [16, 17]. Pathological studies in female radical cystectomy specimens have demonstrated that the urethra is rarely involved in the absence of bladder-neck involvement [18] or extensive carcinoma *in situ* [19]. Preservation of the distal part of the urethral will allow reconstruction of new bladder from the small intestine to be anastomosed to the preserved urethra. Follow up of those patients proved the safety of urethral preservation. This option will definitely increase the acceptance by the patients to do such type of surgery and also will increase its practice among urosurgeons [18–20].

5. Previous reports about genital-sparing cystectomy in patients with urothelial carcinoma

Preservation of the sexual function in women has not been the main goal in most studies of neobladder in women and studies concerning genital-sparing cystectomy are lacking. Only four series were reported addressing this issue; one series of open surgery in three cases of TCC [4], one series of robotic surgery in two cases of TCC [6], one series of laparoscopic surgery in one case of TCC [5], and one series of laparoscopic surgery in 13 cases of neurogenic vesical dysfunction [7]. The number of cases in these studies is limited; the follow up was very short and no report was mentioned on the oncological function in terms of local recurrence (**Table 1**).

Horenblas et al. [4] reported on sexuality preserving cystectomy in three female patients with bladder cancer, using a retrograde method. No patient had a local recurrence, and daytime and nighttime continence was reported in 66% of cases while the remainder needed intermittent catheterization. One patient developed a vaginal urinary fistula and was converted to

http://dx.doi.org/10.5772/67759

Reference	Horenblas et al. [4]	Menon et al. [6]	Game et al. [7]	Moinzadeh et al. [5]	Kulkarni et al. [8]	Koie et al. [9]	Salem [10]
Year	2001	2004	2007	2005	2008	2009	2008
Country	Netherlands	USA	France	USA	India	Japan	Egypt
Pathology	TCC*	TCC	Neurogenic vesical dysfunction	TCC	TCC	29: TCC 1: leiomyosarcoma	TCC
No. of cases	3	3	13	11	14 (retrospective)	30 (retrospective)	20
Genital-sparing cases	3	2	13	1	14	30	20
Technique	Open	Robotic	Laparoscopy	Laparoscopy	Open	Open	Open
Diversion	Orthotopic	Ileal conduit, W pouch, T pouch	Noncontinent trans ileal Bricker	Ileal conduit (8), Studer (2), Indiana pouch (1)	Neobladder	Neobladder (U-shaped)	W pouch (24), Le Bag (1)
Mean op. time (min.)	–	160 (cystectomy) 130 (ileal conduit) 180 (orthotopic)	325 ± 36	510	320	301	210 ± 35
Mean hospital stay	–	6.7	11.6 ± 1.9	6	–	–	11 ± 3
Mean follow-up (months)	3.5	–	7.4 ± 5.4	7.1	32.5	35.7	70
Daytime continence	66%		–	Excellent	7	24	70%
Nighttime continence	66%	–	–	Excellent	7	24	85%
Hypercontinence (intermittent catheterization)	33%	–	–	−ve	4	0	15%
Local recurrence	−ve	–	–	–	1	1	0%
Mean blood loss (cc)	–	100	343.1 ± 246.3	–	300–1500	983	300 ± 120

Table 1. Showing previous reports on genital-sparing cystectomy.

a continent catheterizable stoma. Vaginal lubrication and orgasmic feeling were reported to be normal after surgery.

Menon et al. [6] reported robotic-assisted radical cystectomy in three female patients, one of them was anterior exenteration and two of them genital-sparing cystectomy. No report was mentioned on the mean follow up, continence, or local recurrence.

In our previous study, we excluded the pathology of the internal genitalia by standard clinical and gynecological examination. To decrease the risk of subsequent local recurrence, we excluded patients with tumor at the trigone, posterior wall, bladder neck, and associated carcinoma *in situ*. For greater safety, we did intraoperative frozen section biopsy of the urethral surgical margin. The surgical margins were free in all patients (urethral margin, posterior bladder wall). Only in one case, there was microscopic invasion of the anterior wall (pT3a III TCC). At the last follow up, all patients are alive and well with no evidence of disease recurrence. None of these had urethral or vaginal recurrences. Seventeen (85%) patients voided spontaneously. Fourteen (70%) of them were continent day and night and three of them suffering from some form of urge or stress incontinence in the first 3 months after surgery. The remaining three patients (15%) needed regular self-catheterization (hyper continent). Median bladder capacity at the last follow up was 450 cc (350–600). Median residual urine was 100 cc (0–350). All patients were sexually active 3 months after surgery. Vaginal lubrication was reported in 16 patients. Two patients were suffering from dyspareunia. Orgasmic function was preserved in 16 patients [10].

6. Value of preservation of the internal genital organs in female patients undergoing radical cystectomy

There is no doubt that removal of the internal genitalia in premenopausal women will affect the quality of life of such patient and will cause psychological trauma especially in young patients eager to have children. With increasing survival from urologic cancer, quality of life, and quality of sexuality should be one of the main goals following radical cystectomy in female patients with bladder cancer. Hence, routine removal of the internal genitalia has to be investigated thoroughly.

Preservation of the internal gynecological organs will improve the functional outcome and will have positive impact on the quality of life after exclusion of concomitant primary or secondary gynecological malignancy by careful preoperative assessment.

6.1. The vagina

The preserved vagina will provide backing to the neobladder, prevent pouchocele formation in the dead space, provide better support to the distal urethra to prevent kinking of the urethropouch anastomosis decreasing the likelihood of hyper continence, and maintain the sexual function in women who want it particularly if nerve-sparing technique was done and vaginal lubrication was preserved. No chance of fistula formation between the vagina and the new pouch because there is no suture line in the preserved vagina.

http://dx.doi.org/10.5772/67759

In patients with urothelial carcinoma away from the bladder base or the bladder neck (dome and anterior wall tumors), the anterior vaginal wall may be preserved [21]. The oncological safety of preservation of the anterior vaginal wall has been proved in another study by Chen et al. in 1996 in a retrospective study at MD Anderson Cancer Center [22].

6.2. The uterus

The uterus will retain the reproductive function in this group of patients, in addition, the uterus will prevent vaginal vault or pelvic prolapse. Chang et al. [23] suggested that preservation of uterus and its supports may prevent the dead space that otherwise would be filled by small bowel which in some may produce anterior enterocele following cystectomy as was reported by Anderson et al. [24]. The uterus also plays a role in orgasmic function [25].

Removal of the uterus may be associated with psychological trauma in young sexually active women eager to have a child when future pregnancy is contemplated.

We believe that in postmenopausal women or in those who no longer desire future fertility, hysterectomy seems a reasonable adjunct to cystectomy.

6.3. The ovaries

Data concerning metastasis of bladder TCC to the ovaries are scarce and autopsy studies showed that ovarian metastasis due to TCC of the bladder ranged between 0 and 9% [26–29]. Marshall and Treiger suggested one ovary to be left to preserve the hormonal function after radical cystectomy [30], acute premature menopause (ovarian hormone deprivation) is associated with increased menopausal symptoms, ischemic heart disease, and osteoporosis risk. Prolonged hormone replacement therapy used to alleviate symptoms and minimize these risks has been associated with increased incidence of breast cancer especially if used for more than 5 years [31].

The criteria for patients selection for genital sparing include the following: single monofocal localized tumor, away from the bladder neck, trigone or posterior wall, no associated carcinoma *in situ*, patient with serum creatinine of less than 1.7 mg/dl, patient agree and able to perform self-catheterization, patient motivated for preservation of sexual function (sexually active), and no cervical or uterine abnormalities.

7. Conclusion

Here, we have described a technique of genital-sparing radical cystectomy with orthotopic neobladder in selected female patients. The technique is feasible and of low morbidity with reasonable oncological and functional outcome. Although radical cystectomy is the gold standard for female patients with bladder cancer, preservation of the internal genitalia in young sexually active women eager to have children should be considered in selected cases under strict criteria. The desire to achieve functional good results should not violate the oncological surgical principles.

Author details

Hosni Khairy Salem

Address all correspondence to: dr_hosni@yahoo.com

Urology Department, Faculty of Medicine, Kasr Alainy Hospital, Cairo University, Cairo, Egypt

References

[1] Stein JP, Ginsberg DA and Skinner DG: Indications and technique of the orthotopic neobladder in women. Urol Clin North Am. 2002; 29: 725–4.

[2] Stein JP, Grossfeld GD, Freeman JA, Esrig D, Ginsberg GA, Cote RJ et al.: Orthotopic lower urinary tract reconstruction in women using the Kock ilealneobladder: updated experience in 34 patients. J Urol. 1997; 158: 400–5.

[3] Shimogaki H, Okada H, Fujisawa M, Arakawa S, Kawabata G, Kamidono S et al.: Long-term experience with orthotopic reconstruction of the lower urinary tract in women. J Urol. 1999; 161: 573–7.

[4] Horenblas S, Meinhardt W, Lizerman W and Moonen LF: Sexuality preserving cystectomy and neobladder: initial results. J Urol. 2001; 166: 837–40.

[5] Moinzadeh A, Gill I, Desai M, Finelli A, Falconi T and Jihad J: Laparoscopic radical cystectomy in the female. J Urol. 2005; 173: 1912–17.

[6] Menon M, Hemal AK, Tewari A, Shrivastava A, Shoma AM, Abol-Ein H, et al.: Robot-assisted radical cystectomy and urinary diversion in female patients: technique with preservation of the uterus and vagina. JACS. 2004; 198: 386–93.

[7] Game X, Mallet R, Guillotreau J, Berrogain N, Mouzin M, et al.: Uterus, fallopian tube, ovary and vagina-spring laparoscopic cystectomy: technical description and results. Eur Urol. 2007; 51: 441–46.

[8] Kulkarni JN, Rizni SJ, Acharya UP, Kumar KS and Tiwari P: Gynecologic-tract sparing extraperitoneal retrograde radical cystectomy with neobladder. Int Braz J Urol. 2008; 34: 180–90.

[9] Koie T, Hatakeyama S, Yoneyama T, Hashimoto Y, Kamimura N, and Ohyama C: Uterus, fallopian tube, ovary, and vaginal—sparing cystectomy followed by U-shaped ileal neobladder construction for female bladder cancer patients: oncological and functional outcome. Urol. 2010; 75: 1499–1503.

[10] Salem H: Functional and oncological outcome of genital-sparing radical cystectomy in female patients with muscle invasive transitional cell carcinoma (TCC) of the bladder. JOU. 2008; 179(4): 239. DOI: 10.1016/S0022-5347(08)60852-6.

[11] Groutz A, Gillon G, Konichezky M, Shimonov M, Winkler H, Livne PM et al.: Involvement of internal genitalia in female patients undergoing radical, cystectomy for bladder cancer: a clinicopathologic study of 37 cases. Int J Gynecol Cancer. 1999; 9: 302–6.

[12] Chang SS, Cole E, Smith JA Jr, Cookson MS: Pathological findings of gynecologic organs obtained at female radical cystectomy. J Urol. 2002; 168: 147–9.

[13] Ali-el-Dein B, Abdel-Latif M, Mosbah A, Eraky I, Shabaan AA, Taha N M et al.: Secondary malignant involvement of gynecologic organs in radical cystectomy specimens in women: is it mandatory to remove these organs routinely? J Urol. 2004; 172: 885–7.

[14] Hosni Salem, Akmal El-Mazny: Primary and secondary malignant involvement of gynaecological organs at radical cystectomy for bladder cancer: review of literature and retrospective analysis of 360 cases. J Obstet Gynaecol. 2012, 32(6):590–3. DOI: 10.3109/01443615.2012.693980.

[15] Salem H, El-Mazny A: Aclinico pathological study off gynecological organs involvement in radical cystectomy for bladder cancer. Int J Gynecol Obstet. 2011; 115: 188–190.

[16] Coloby PJ, Kakizoe T, Tobisu K and Sakamoto M: Urethral involvement in female bladder cancer patients: mapping of 47 consecutive cystourethrectomy specimens. J Urol. 1994; 152: 1438–42.

[17] Stenzle A, Draxl H, Posch B, Colleselli K, Falk M and Bartsch G: The risk of urethral tumors in female bladder cancer: can the urethra be used for orthotopic reconstruction of the lower urinary tract? J Urol. 1995; 153: 950–5.

[18] Stein JP, Cote RJ, Freeman JA, Esrig D, Elmajian DA, Groshen S et al.: Indications for lower urinary tract reconstruction in women after cystectomy for bladder cancer: a pathological review of female cystectomy specimens. J Urol. 1995; 154: 1329–33.

[19] Stein JP, Esrig D, Freeman JA, GrossfeldGD, Ginsberg GA, Cote RJ et al.: Prospective pathologic analysis of female cystectomy specimens: risk factors for orthotopic diversion in women. Urol. 1998; 51: 951–5.

[20] Stenzl A, Jarolim L, Coloby P, Golia S, Bartsch G, Babjuk M et al.: Urethra-sparing cystectomy and orthotopic urinary diversion in women with malignant pelvic tumors. Cancer. 2001; 92: 1864–71

[21] Freiha FS: Open bladder surgery. In: Walsh PC, Retik AB, Stamey TA, Caghan ED, eds. Campbell's Urology. New York: W.B. Saunders; p. 2762, 1992.

[22] Chen ME, Malpica A, Dinney CP and Pisters LL: Risk of urethral, vaginal and cervical involvement in patients undergoing radical cystectomy for bladder cancer: a retrospective review of patients at M.D Anderson Cancer Center. AUA Ninety-first Annual Meeting. J. Urol. 1996; 155: 1263 (Abstract).

[23] Chang SS, Cole E, Cookson MS, Peterson M and Smith JA Jr.: Preservation of the anterior vaginal wall during female radical cystectomy with orthotopic urinary diversion: technique and results. J Urol. 2002; 168: 1442–5.

[24] Anderson J, Carrion R, Ordorica R, Hoffman M, Arango H and Lockhart JL: Anterior enterocele following cystectomy for intractable interstitial cystitis. J Urol. 1998; 159: 1868–70.

[25] Weijmar Schultz WC, Van De Wiel HB, Hahn DE and Bouma J: Psychosexual functioning after treatment for gynecological cancer: an integrative model, review of determinant factors and clinical guidelines. Int J Gynecol Cancer. 1992; 2: 281–90.

[26] Babaian RJ, Johnson DE, Llamas L and Ayala AG: Metastases from transitional cell carcinoma of the urinary bladder. Urol. 1980; 16: 142–4.

[27] Fetter TR, Bogaer JH, McCuskey B and Seres JL: Carcinoma of the bladder: sites of metastases. J Urol. 1959; 81: 746–8.

[28] Kishi K, Hirota T, Matsumoto K, Kakizoe T, Murase T and Fujita J: Carcinoma of the bladder: a clinical and pathological analysis of 87 autopsy cases. J Urol. 1981; 125: 36–9.

[29] Murphy GP: The current status of bladder cancer. Surg Ann. 1975; 7: 175–218.

[30] Marshall FF and Treiger BFG: Radical cystectomy in the female patient. Urol Clin North Am. 1991, 18: 765–70.

[31] Colditz GA, Hankinson SE, Hunter DJ et al.: The use of estrogens and progestins and the risk of breast cancer in postmenopausal women. N Engl J Med. 1995; 332: 1589–93.